T0252863

Yoga and Anatomy

An Experiential Atlas of Movement

Barbie Klein, PhD
Assistant Professor
Department of Anatomy
University of California
San Francisco, California, USA

Mackenzie Loyet, MA, MS, RYT 200
Anatomy Instructor and Laboratory Coordinator
Department of Anatomy
Midwestern University
Downers Grove, Illinois, USA

207 illustrations

Anatomical illustrations in Part II by Voll M and Wesker K. from resp. based on: Schuenke M, Schulte E, Schumacher U, THIEME Atlas of Anatomy

Thieme
New York • Stuttgart • Delhi • Rio de Janeiro

Library of Congress Cataloging-in-Publication Data is available from the publisher

Important note: Medicine is an ever-changing science undergoing continual development. Research and clinical experience are continually expanding our knowledge, in particular our knowledge of proper treatment and drug therapy. Insofar as this book mentions any dosage or application, readers may rest assured that the authors, editors, and publishers have made every effort to ensure that such references are in accordance with the state of **knowledge at the time of production of the book.**

Nevertheless, this does not involve, imply, or express any guarantee or responsibility on the part of the publishers in respect to any dosage instructions and forms of applications stated in the book. **Every user is requested to examine carefully** the manufacturers' leaflets accompanying each drug and to check, if necessary in consultation with a physician or specialist, whether the dosage schedules mentioned therein or the contraindications stated by the manufacturers differ from the statements made in the present book. Such examination is particularly important with drugs that are either rarely used or have been newly released on the market. Every dosage schedule or every form of application used is entirely at the user's own risk and responsibility. The authors and publishers request every user to report to the publishers any discrepancies or inaccuracies noticed. If errors in this work are found after publication, errata will be posted at www.thieme.com on the product description page.

Some of the product names, patents, and registered designs referred to in this book are in fact registered trademarks or proprietary names even though specific reference to this fact is not always made in the text. Therefore, the appearance of a name without designation as proprietary is not to be construed as a representation by the publisher that it is in the public domain.

©2020. Thieme. All rights reserved.

Thieme Publishers New York
333 Seventh Avenue, New York, NY 10001 USA
+1 800 782 3488, customerservice@thieme.com

Georg Thieme Verlag KG
Rüdigerstrasse 14, 70469 Stuttgart, Germany
+49 [0]711 8931 421, customerservice@thieme.de

Thieme Publishers Delhi
A-12, Second Floor, Sector-2, Noida-201301
Uttar Pradesh, India
+91 120 45 566 00, customerservice@thieme.in

Thieme Publishers Rio de Janeiro,
Thieme Publicações Ltda.
Edifício Rodolpho de Paoli, 25º andar
Av. Nilo Peçanha, 50 – Sala 2508,
Rio de Janeiro 20020-906 Brasil
+55 21 3172-2297

Cover design: Thieme Publishing Group
Typesetting by Thomson Digital, India

Printed in USA by King Printing Company, Inc.

ISBN 978-1-62623-830-5

Also available as an e-book:
eISBN 978-1-62623-832-9

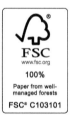

This book, including all parts thereof, is legally protected by copyright. Any use, exploitation, or commercialization outside the narrow limits set by copyright legislation, without the publisher's consent, is illegal and liable to prosecution. This applies in particular to photostat reproduction, copying, mimeographing, preparation of microfilms, and electronic data processing and storage.

Disclaimer: Please consult physician prior to beginning yoga. The authors of this book cannot be held responsible for any injury sustained while practicing yoga.

Contents

Preface

In 2014, as graduate students in an anatomy education program, we investigated better ways to teach the musculoskeletal system to our students. It may be tempting to think that memorizing muscle names and locations is the only way to learn the material in your anatomy course; however, modern theories of teaching and learning have found that active engagement and deliberate practice support knowledge acquisition and the development of expertise.[1,2] Experiential learning occurs when learners are engaged and construct knowledge through practical, real-world applications followed by a period of time to reflect on their learning.[3] Since we both practiced yoga, it seemed logical to combine the idea of experiential learning in the context of yoga practice. Inspired by previous studies on kinesthetic learning,[4,5] we developed a yoga/anatomy workshop for our students in order to review the musculoskeletal system through the movement of yoga poses (*asanas*). Yoga is an ideal medium for exploring the role of muscular function, as poses can be moved through slowly (allowing time to explain muscle functions) and linked together with breath to create a yoga flow (*vinyasa*). During our workshops, we guided students into an *asana* while we explained the actions at joints, drawing their attention to the muscular sensations (such as stretching and contracting) that they were feeling. This workshop encouraged students to connect class material to physical movements and further promoted body awareness. It was during the course of these yoga/anatomy workshops that the idea for this atlas was born.

Many books focusing on yoga and anatomy today illustrate the musculoskeletal system only in the final, static posture. One of the goals of this book is to explain how to safely enter and exit a specific yoga pose and highlight the various muscular transitions involved. Furthermore, we wanted to emphasize the movements of joints and innervations of muscles, as students move from one transitional pose to the next. Body and breath awareness is the foundational aspect of yoga, and we hope that this atlas will help you connect your own anatomy to your personal yoga practice.

Many muscles contract simultaneously to produce a singular action. To manage cognitive load[6] and enhance the educational value of this atlas, we decided to highlight specific muscles for each pose sequence. Although muscles are shown in isolation, the atlas has endeavored to spread awareness about the fact that multiple muscles work simultaneously to complete movements; therefore, we focus on the movements of major joints as you flow between each transition. While we aimed for anatomical accuracy in each progressive pose, artistic compromises were considered, so bear in mind that every muscle described in the text is not drawn on all figures and images. We encourage you to use Part II of this atlas as a reference to better understand the muscle's origin, insertion, and its anatomical relationship to other structures in the body. In addition, physiologic and kinesiologic principles are considered outside the scope of this atlas; thus, all muscular functions are discussed as concentric contractions (rather than eccentric and isometric contractions). Also, we have referred to "stretching" as the lengthening of muscles, and "contraction" as the active shortening of muscle fibers which act on bones to produce movements at joints.

We hope that you find this resource helpful in understanding the musculoskeletal system and how the body moves during yoga practice. Designed for individuals who are beginners to yoga, we encourage you to connect anatomy with both your everyday movements and yoga postures. For students of anatomy, we feel that this book will make an excellent supplemental text to your other anatomy resources. We would appreciate your comments and feedback.

Namaste.

Barbie Klein, PhD
Mackenzie Loyet, MA, MS, RYT 200

References

1. Garbarini F, Adenzato M. At the root of embodied cognition: cognitive science meets neurophysiology. Brain Cogn 2004;56:100–106.
2. Kolb D. Experiential Learning: Experience as the source of Learning and Development. 2nd ed. Upper Saddle River, NJ: Pearson FT Press 2014.
3. Yardley S, Teunissen PW, Dornan T. Experiential learning: transforming theory into practice. Med Teach 2012;34:161–164.
4. Bentley D, Pang, S. Yoga asanas as an effective form of experiential learning when teaching musculoskeletal anatomy of the lower limb. Anat Sci Educ 2012;5:281–286.
5. McCulloch C, Marango S, Friedman E, Laitman J. Living AnatoME: teaching and learning musculoskeletal anatomy through yoga and pilates. Anat Sci Educ 2010;3:279–286.
6. Khalil M, Paas F, Johnson T, Payer A. Design of interactive and dynamic anatomical visualizations: the implication of cognitive load theory. Anat Rec 2005;286:15–20.

Acknowledgments

We would like to extend our sincerest gratitude to our academic adviser, Dr. Valerie O'Loughlin, who was instrumental in developing our original yoga/anatomy workshops. We would like to convey our thanks to our students who participated in the evolution and development of this project. This atlas would not have been possible without the wonderful work and patience of our model, Bridget Hayes. We would also like to thank our Thieme editors, Delia DeTurris and Prakash Naorem. Finally, a very special thank you to Brenda Bunch and Rebecca Symonds (also from Thieme) for all the medical illustrations of Part I in the book.

Barbie Klein, PhD
Mackenzie Loyet, MA, MS, RYT 200

How to Use this Atlas

As you read through this atlas, note that the yoga poses in Part I are divided into seven different categories by chapter: standing poses, standing balancing poses, forward folds, backbends, arm balances, spinal twists, and inversions. Each chapter illustrates three to four different *asanas* (postures) and the transitions involved to reach the final expression of the poses. For every pose, we include the Sanskrit and the English names and discuss modifications (use of props such as blocks and a strap).

In the yoga pose descriptions, we provide references to figures or tables in Part II of the book to help you visualize muscle locations, orientations, and remind you of important information, such as actions of muscles and their innervations.

Please note that only the muscles in the final expression of the pose are drawn. To aid in visualizing surface anatomy, muscles in all the other pose transitions are indicated by arrows: a grey arrow represents a contracting muscle and a teal arrow represents a stretching muscle. Finally, muscles that are deep or cannot be easily seen from a particular view are indicated with an asterisk.

We encourage you to listen to your body, move with intention, and only transition to the final expression of a pose when you feel comfortable in the preparatory poses.

Part I

Yoga Poses
(Asanas)

1   Standing Poses

Chair
(Utkatasana)

Summary of the Pose

Translated as "Awkward or Ferocious Pose", this standing posture resembles sitting toward the back of a chair and strengthens the muscles of the core, hip flexors, and hamstrings.

Modifications: Bring your palms to touch overhead and look up for an additional neck stretch. Place a block between your thighs to promote internal rotation of both femurs. If you experience shoulder pain, practice this pose with both hands at your sternum.

Guided Narrative

Transition 1: Mountain

- Begin in anatomical position by standing with feet hips-width distance apart, aligned directly under your pelvic bones.
- Press evenly through both calcanei and the heads of all five metatarsals.
- Use supinator (**Fig. 10.13**) in both forearms to rotate your palms anteriorly.
- Your ascending fibers of trapezius (**Fig. 10.7**) work to depress the scapulae and draw your scapulae down your back.
- Engage your quadriceps femoris (**Fig. 11.1**) to lift your patellae proximally.
- Tighten your core and use your abdominal muscles (**Fig. 9.5**) to draw in your umbilicus and stabilize your trunk.

●●

Transition 2: Upward Hand

- Inhale and abduct your arms overhead, using supraspinatus and deltoid (**Fig. 10.2**).
- Engage the transverse part of your trapezius to draw your scapulae medially retracting your scapulae. Your rhomboid major and rhomboid minor (**Fig. 10.8**) will also contribute to this medial movement of your scapulae.
- Rotate your palms to face each other, using your infraspinatus and teres minor muscles of the rotator cuff (**Fig. 10.4**) to laterally rotate the humerus.
- Note that your radial nerve assists with extension through your elbows, wrists, and fingers by innervating the muscles of the posterior compartments of your arm and forearm.

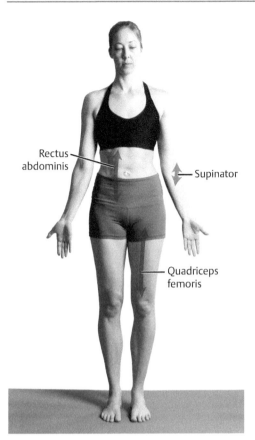

Rectus abdominis

Supinator

Quadriceps femoris

Transition 1: **Mountain**

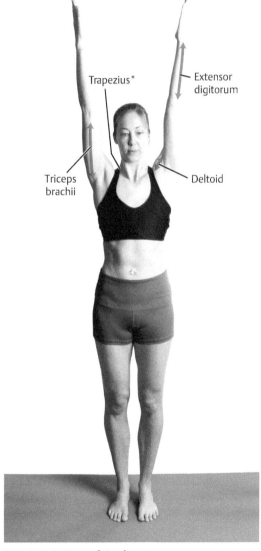

Trapezius*

Extensor digitorum

Triceps brachii

Deltoid

Transition 2: **Upward Hand**

Final Pose: **Chair**

- While maintaining the extension of the upper body using triceps brachii (**Fig. 10.11**) and the muscles of the posterior compartment of your forearm, begin to flex both hip and knee joints and sit back. Feel rectus femoris, sartorius, and tensor fasciae latae (**Fig. 11.1**) flexing at the hip joints while your hamstrings (**Fig. 11.4**) flex both knees.
- Engage your adductor muscles to draw your knees together while gluteus medius (**Fig. 11.4**) helps to internally rotate the hips.
- Rock weight into the calcanei of both feet. Option to extend all ten toes off the mat to challenge your balance and feel the dorsiflexors of the anterior compartment of the leg contracting, and then release your toes back to the mat.
- On both arms lifted, the inferior part of serratus anterior (**Fig. 10.6**) is working to upwardly rotate your scapulae.
- On every inhalation, work on reaching your fingers higher toward the ceiling while continuing to depress your scapulae. Sit back further with every exhalation, flexing more at the knees (as is comfortable).
- Extend your knees and hips, then lower your arms back into anatomical position to release from this pose.

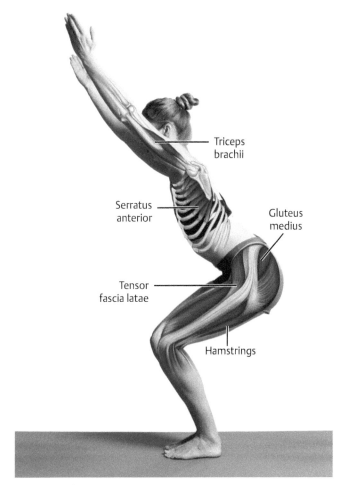

Triceps
brachii

Serratus
anterior

Gluteus
medius

Tensor
fascia latae

Hamstrings

Final Pose: **Chair**

Warrior I
(Virabhadrasana I)

Summary of the Pose

Named after the Sanskrit word *vira*, meaning hero, this is a foundational pose in yoga that strengthens the ankles, calves, hips, abdominals, and low back.

Modifications: If you experience shoulder pain, press your palms together anterior to your sternum. You may also shorten the distance between your front and back foot to decrease the intensity of the hip stretch.

Guided Narrative

Transition 1: **Forward Fold**

- From anatomical position, with your feet together or hips-width distance apart, contract your abdominals (**Fig. 9.7**) to flex your vertebral column and fold at your hips bringing your chest toward your thighs.
- Place your hands on the mat; if the ground seems far away, flex your knees or place your palms on blocks.
- Lift your patellae proximally by contracting quadriceps femoris (**Fig. 11.1**) to feel a deep stretch across your hamstrings (**Fig. 11.1**).
- Relax your head and neck and gaze between your legs. Only go as a deep in this fold as you are comfortable.
- As you press into the mat or blocks, notice triceps brachii (**Fig. 10.10**) working to extend your elbows.

• •

Transition 2: **Low Lunge**

- Use your left hamstrings and gluteus maximus (**Fig. 11.8**) to extend your thigh placing your left foot near the back of your mat.
- Ensure that the patella of your right knee is aligned superior to your right ankle.
- Contract your abdominals to flex your vertebral column and draw your umbilicus up and in, away from your right thigh.
- Bilaterally contract trapezius supplied by the spinal accessory nerve (cranial nerve XI), splenius capitis, and longissimus capitis (**Fig. 8.2**) to slightly extend your head and neck to gaze a few inches in front of your mat.
- As you push into the ground, feel serratus anterior (**Fig. 10.6**) protract your scapulae and notice that deltoid and the muscles of the rotator cuff (**Fig. 10.4**) help to stabilize the shoulder joint.

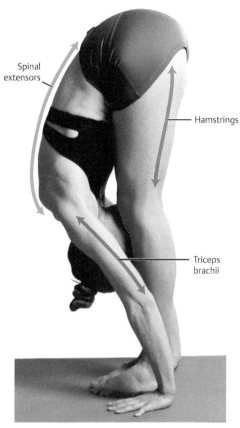

Spinal extensors

Hamstrings

Triceps brachii

Transition 1: **Forward Fold**

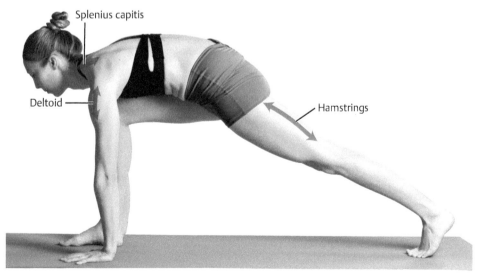

Splenius capitis

Deltoid

Hamstrings

Transition 2: **Low Lunge**

Final Pose: **Warrior I**

- On an inhalation, rotate your back foot to about a 45-degree angle and bring yourself up by ipsilaterally contracting your left abdominal obliques (**Fig. 9.7**) and erector spinae to laterally flex your torso.
- Engage quadriceps femoris in your back left leg to extend your left knee. Maintain the flexion in your right knee and knee above ankle alignment from Low Lunge.
- Use your adductors, including gracilis (**Fig. 11.3**), to adduct both thighs toward the midline.
- Inhale and flex both arms overhead, utilizing the clavicular part of deltoid (innervated by the axillary nerve) and biceps brahii (innervated by the musculocutaneous nerve). Feel a stretch in your abdominal obliques.
- The middle and ascending fibers of trapezius work to draw both scapulae medially and downward (**Fig. 10.7**) while triceps brachii extends your forearms. Point your fingers toward the ceiling by contracting extensor digitorum.
- On an exhalation, step your left foot to meet your right at the top of the mat and repeat this sequence on the other side.

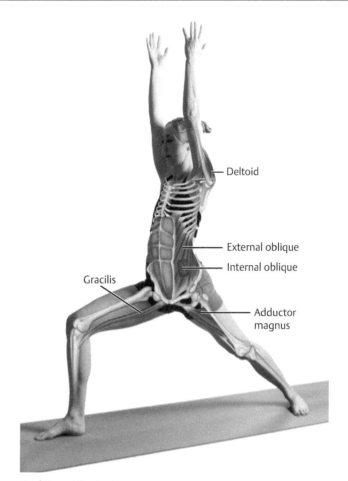

Deltoid

External oblique

Internal oblique

Gracilis

Adductor magnus

Final Pose: **Warrior I**

Warrior II
(Virabhadrasana II)

Summary of the Pose

Named after a warrior scouting out their prey, this standing pose stretches the muscles and ligaments around the hip joints as well as the muscles across the chest and shoulders.

Modifications: Individuals with neck pain should avoid rotating their head in this pose. If maintaining your balance while standing in this pose is challenging, try Warrior II while seated at the edge of a chair for support.

Guided Narrative

Transition 1: **Three-legged Down Dog**

- From Downward Facing Dog, use gluteus maximus and the hamstrings (**Fig. 11.4**) to extend your right thigh at the hip, lifting your right leg into the air.
- Push your palms into the mat and feel serratus anterior protracting your scapulae and trapezius (**Fig. 10.7**) depressing your scapulae, creating space between the ears and shoulders.
- Feel both quadriceps femoris (**Fig. 11.1**) extend your knees and a stretch across the muscles of the posterior compartment of your grounded left leg.
- Use tibialis anterior (**Fig. 11.14**) to dorsiflex your right foot and angle your toes toward the ground to help internally rotate your right hip.

• •

Transition 2: **Knee to Nose**

- Bring your patella toward the nose using psoas major and iliacus (**Fig. 9.6**) to flex your right thigh at the hip and your hamstrings to flex your right knee. Shift forward so that your shoulders stack superior to the wrists.
- Note that triceps brachii are working to extend both elbows (**Fig. 10.11**). Abduct through the fingers using your dorsal interossei (**Fig. 10.15**) creating a wide base for this arm balance.
- Contract rectus abdominis (**Fig. 9.5**) to flex your vertebral column and draw the umbilicus up and into the core.
- Plantarflex your right foot at the ankle, feeling the contraction of gastrocnemius and soleus (**Fig. 11.16**).

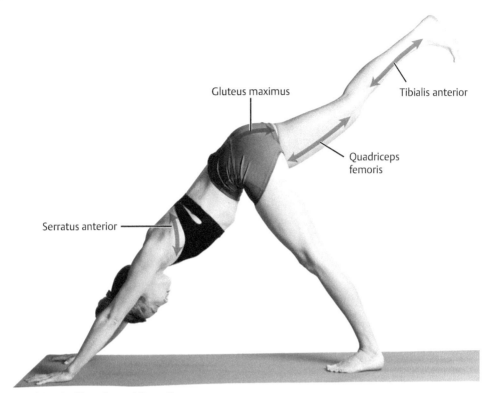

Gluteus maximus

Tibialis anterior

Quadriceps femoris

Serratus anterior

Transition 1: **Three-Legged Down Dog**

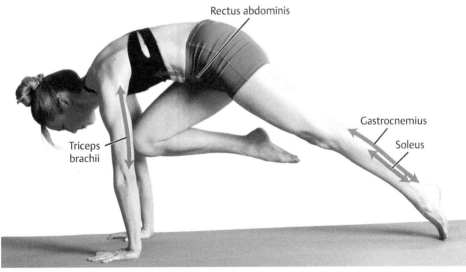

Rectus abdominis

Gastrocnemius

Soleus

Triceps brachii

Transition 2: **Knee to Nose**

Transition 3: **Low Lunge**

- Slowly contract quadriceps femoris to extend your right leg, placing the plantar surface of the right foot to the ground between the palms.
- Ensure that the patella of your right knee is aligned superior to your ankle.
- Contract your abdominals to flex your vertebral column and draw your umbilicus up and in, away from your right thigh.
- Bilaterally contract trapezius, splenius capitis, and longissimus capitis (**Fig. 9.2**) to slightly extend your head at the neck to gaze a few inches in front of your mat.
- As you push into the ground, feel serratus anterior (**Fig. 10.6**) protract your scapulae and stability of your shoulder joints from deltoid and the muscles of the rotator cuff (**Fig. 10.4**).
- Notice that your hamstrings (**Fig. 11.4**), supplied by the tibial nerve and common fibular nerve, and gluteus maximus (**Fig. 11.8**), supplied by the inferior gluteal nerve, are working to extend your left thigh at the hip.

Final Pose: **Warrior II**

- Rotate your left foot to place the plantar surface to the ground, aligning the lateral edge of your back foot parallel to the back edge of the mat. Notice that the lateral rotators of the hip (**Fig. 11.9**) assist with this action and both hips are now externally rotated.
- Align the calcaneus of your right foot with the arch of the left foot.
- To rise vertically, laterally flex your torso by ipsilaterally contracting your left obliques, erector spinae, and quadratus lumborum (**Fig. 9.7**).
- Use supraspinatus and deltoid to abduct your arms out to the sides as you lift into Warrior II.
- Align your arms and forearms parallel to the floor with palms facing down and stack your shoulder joints superior to your hip joints. Extend the elbows, wrists, and digits.
- Briefly look down at your front foot, you should be able to see your hallux. If not, externally rotate your thigh to move your knee laterally until your knee stacks above the ankle.
- Engage your right psoas major to maintain flexion of the front hip. Notice that your right hamstrings are flexing your front knee and your left quadriceps femoris extends the back knee.
- Your left sternocleidomastoid and right splenius (**Fig. 9.1**) contract to turn your head to the right, gazing past the third distal phalanx.
- With every inhale, extend your vertebral column and with every exhale, sink deeper into your front lunge.
- Exhale to low lunge and then step your right foot back to meet your left in Downward Facing Dog. Repeat this sequence on the left side.

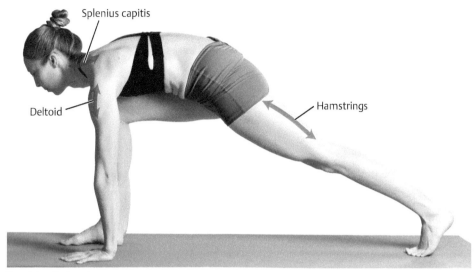

Splenius capitis

Deltoid

Hamstrings

Transition 3: **Low Lunge**

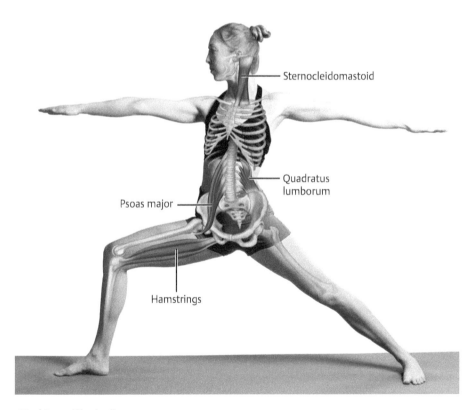

Sternocleidomastoid

Quadratus lumborum

Psoas major

Hamstrings

Final Pose: **Warrior II**

Triangle
(Utthita Trikonasana)

Summary of the Pose

This pose incorporates both movements of grounding and lifting. It stretches the inner thighs and chest, as well as strengthens the thighs and core.

Modifications: Option to bring a block under the bottom hand or to keep a microbend in the front knee. Do not turn your head to look up if you experience any neck pain.

Guided Narrative

Transition 1: **Warrior II**

- From standing, use gluteus medius and gluteus minimus (**Fig. 11.4**) to abduct your left hip and step your feet wide. Ensure that the calcaneus of your right foot is aligned with the middle of the arch of the left foot.
- Rotate your left foot to place the plantar surface to the ground, aligning the lateral edge of your back foot parallel to the back edge of the mat. Notice that the lateral rotators of the hip (**Fig. 11.9**) assist with this action and both hips are now externally rotated.
- Briefly look down at your front foot. You should be able to see your hallux; if not, externally rotate your thigh to move your knee laterally.
- Notice that your right hamstrings (**Fig. 11.4**) are flexing your front knee and your left quadriceps femoris (**Fig. 11.1**) extends the back knee.
- Feel supraspinatus and deltoid abduct your arms out to the sides so that your arms and forearms are parallel to the floor with palms facing down.
- Stack your shoulder joints above the hip joints and extend your elbows, wrists, and digits.
- Gaze past your right third distal phalanx by contracting your left sternocleidomastoid and right splenius capitis (**Fig. 9.1**) to revolve your head to the right.

• •

Transition 2: **Extended Side Angle**

- Laterally flex your torso to the right by ipsilaterally contracting your right internal and external obliques, erector spinae, and quadratus lumborum (**Fig. 9.7**).
- Place your right palm to the ground or to a block medial to your right foot. Alternatively, place your right forearm on your thigh.
- Feel deltoid (**Fig. 10.3**) abduct your left arm at the shoulder, inhaling your hand to the ceiling.
- Turn your gaze up to your left hand using your right sternocleidomastoid and left splenius capitis.
- Lengthen the crown of your head toward the front of the room during your inhalations and twist your torso to the ceiling on your exhalations, moving to stack your left shoulder superior to your right shoulder.

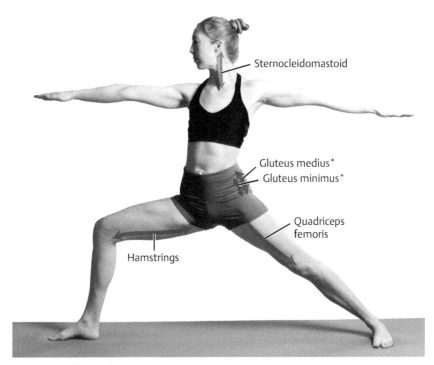

Sternocleidomastoid

Gluteus medius*
Gluteus minimus*

Quadriceps
femoris

Hamstrings

Transition 1: **Warrior II**

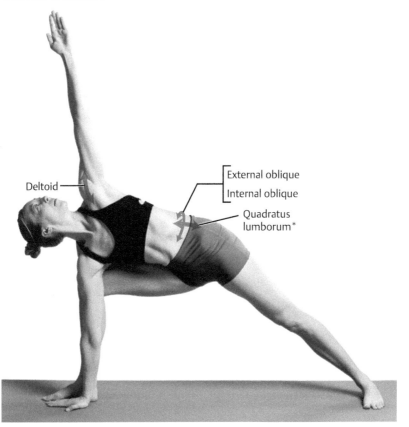

External oblique

Internal oblique

Deltoid

Quadratus
lumborum*

Transition 2: **Extended Side Angle.** Note: To better illustrate the muscles, the left abdominal obliques and quadratus lumborum are indicated on the contralateral side from the guided narrative.

Final Pose: Triangle

- Slowly begin to extend your right leg at the knee activating quadriceps femoris (**Fig. 11.1**).
- Note that your right hip is externally rotated from the action of gluteus maximus, piriformis, and quadratus femoris while the left hip is relatively neutral within the hip joint.
- Feel a stretch across pectoralis major and the clavicular part of your deltoid.
- Triceps brachii (**Fig. 10.11**) work to extend both elbows. Lengthen both sides of your torso evenly and place a block under your right hand for more support if needed.
- Ground down through both feet, gripping the mat using the intrinsic muscles of your feet (**Fig. 11.24**).
- On an inhalation, return upright by laterally flexing your torso using your left internal and external obliques, erector spinae, and quadratus lumborum. Step your left foot to meet your right foot at the top of your mat and repeat the sequence on the other side.

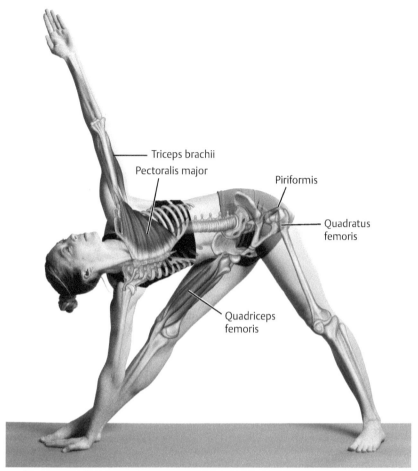

Triceps brachii
Pectoralis major
Piriformis
Quadratus femoris
Quadriceps femoris

Final Pose: Triangle. Note: To better illustrate the muscles, the lateral rotators are indicated on the contralateral side from the guided narrative.

2   Standing Balancing Poses

Tree Pose
(Vrksasana)

Summary of the Pose

This pose improves balance, focus, and patience. It helps strengthen the muscles of the ankles, legs, and arms.

Modifications: Practice this pose holding onto a wall or chair for support until you gain more balance. If healing from a foot injury, use the kickstand variation, described in transition 3, so as not to press all of your weight onto one foot.

Guided Narrative

Transition 1: **One-Legged Mountain**

- From Mountain pose (see chapter 1, standing poses), press your palms together anterior to your sternum and feel trapezius (**Fig. 10.7**) depress and retract your scapulae. Shift weight into the left leg and flex at your right hip to lift the right leg off the floor.
- Continue to engage your hip flexors, including iliacus and psoas major (**Fig. 11.1**) to bring your right knee to the same height as your right hip. Notice that the left hip remains neutral.
- Ensure that your anterior superior iliac spines are both level and pointed forward.
- Dorsiflex the right foot through the innervation of the deep fibular nerve targeting the muscles of the anterior leg (**Fig. 11.14**).
- Lengthen through your vertebral column on your inhalations and engage your abdominal muscles (**Fig. 9.5**) to help maintain balance on your exhalations.

• •

Transition 2: **Tree Prep 1**

- Use piriformis, quadratus femoris, and obturator externus (**Fig. 11.4**) to externally rotate your right hip bringing your right knee out laterally.
- Notice that your right sartorius (**Fig. 11.1**) is also aiding in the lateral rotation of the right thigh.
- Continue to flex your right knee and dorsiflex at your right ankle.
- Engage rectus abdominis to stabilize your core to help maintain the balance.
- Feel the pull of trapezius retract and depress both of your scapulae.

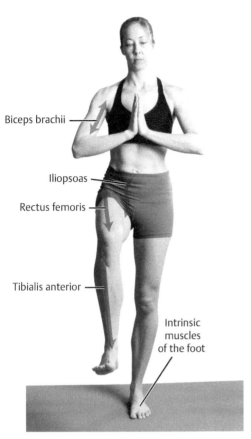

Biceps brachii

Iliopsoas

Rectus femoris

Tibialis anterior

Intrinsic
muscles
of the foot

Transition 1: **One-Legged Mountain**

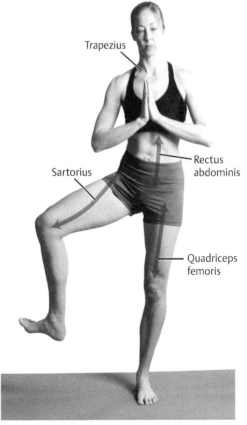

Trapezius

Sartorius

Rectus
abdominis

Quadriceps
femoris

Transition 2: **Tree Prep 1**

Transition 3: **Tree Prep 2**

- While gripping the mat with all four corners of the standing left foot to maintain balance, slowly flex your right knee to rest your right foot on your left leg, either: (1) as a kickstand with right toes on the ground and your heel resting on the standing leg, (2) with the sole of the right foot pressing into the left leg inferior to the knee joint, or (3) with the sole of the right foot pressing into the medial left thigh, superior to the knee joint.
- Avoid placing your right foot directly on the left knee joint.
- Equally press your right foot into your left lower limb as your left lower limb presses back into your right foot. Work toward aligning both your anterior superior iliac spines forward by engaging your sartorius to flex and externally rotate the right hip.
- Focus your gaze *(drishti)* on a single point in front of you that is not moving. For an additional balancing challenge, try lifting your gaze.

· ·

Final Pose: **Tree Pose**

- For the full expression of the pose, begin to "grow your branches" by abducting your shoulders to bring your arms overhead, using supraspinatus and deltoid.
- Triceps brachii are working to extend the elbows here.
- Contract your abdominal muscles to maintain balance and continue to press your right foot firmly into your left lower limb. If you find your right hip dropping, contract the left gluteus medius and gluteus minimus to evenly align your hips in the frontal plane.
- Recall that the dorsiflexion at both ankles is performed by the muscles of the anterior compartment of the leg, including tibialis anterior, extensor digitorum longus, and extensor hallucis longus.
- Try challenging your balance and rely on the proprioception of your joints by closing your eyes.
- Slowly lower your hands back to the sternum and bring your right foot back to the mat. Repeat the pose on the other side.

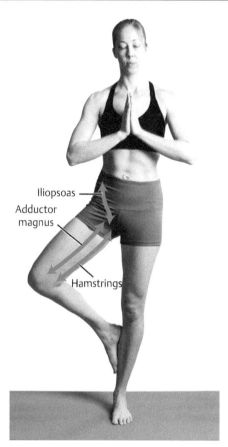

Iliopsoas
Adductor magnus
Hamstrings

Transition 3: **Tree Prep 2**

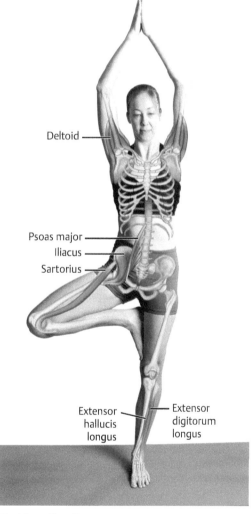

Deltoid

Psoas major
Iliacus
Sartorius

Extensor hallucis longus

Extensor digitorum longus

Final Pose: **Tree Pose**

Warrior III
(Virabhadrasana III)

Summary of the Pose

This pose requires focus and concentration to maintain balance. It helps to strengthen the legs, thighs, back, and core.

Modifications: Bring your hands to blocks or a wall for a supported variation or place the lifted foot on a chair behind you to help with balance.

Guided Narrative

Transition 1: **Low Lunge**

- Start in low lunge with your right foot forward. Feel the extension through your back left thigh from the action of your hamstrings and gluteus maximus (**Fig. 11.4**).
- Ensure that the patella of your right knee is aligned superior to your ankle.
- Contract your abdominals to flex your vertebral column and draw your umbilicus up and in, away from your right thigh.
- Bilaterally contract trapezius supplied by the spinal accessory nerve (cranial nerve XI), splenius capitis, and longissimus capitis (**Fig. 8.2**) to slightly extend your head at the neck to gaze a few inches in front of your mat.
- As you push into the ground, feel serratus anterior (**Fig. 10.6**) protract your scapulae and utilize your deltoid and muscles of the rotator cuff (**Fig. 10.4**) to stabilize your shoulder joints.

•••

Transition 2: **High Lunge**

- On an inhalation, lift your upper body to a vertical position feeling erector spinae (**Fig. 8.3**) extend your vertebral column.
- Abduct your arms using supraspinatus and deltoid (**Fig. 10.2**) to bring your hands above your head. Extend your forearms parallel to each other using triceps brachii and anconeus (**Fig. 10.11**).
- Visualize the ascending fibers of trapezius (**Fig. 10.7**) as they work to depress your scapulae.
- On an exhalation, deepen your lunge by reengaging your right hamstrings to flex your front leg and feel your left quadriceps femoris extend your back leg.
- Draw your right hip back and left hip forward to square your anterior superior iliac spines to the front of the room.

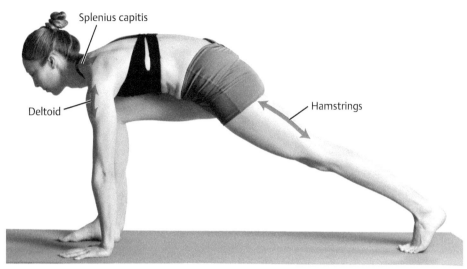

Splenius capitis

Deltoid

Hamstrings

Transition 1: **Low Lunge**

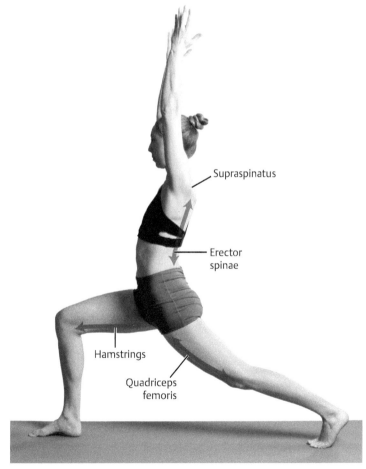

Supraspinatus

Erector spinae

Hamstrings

Quadriceps femoris

Transition 2: **High Lunge**

Final Pose: **Warrior III**

- Shift forward and evenly distribute your weight into your right foot by activating the intrinsic muscles within the foot (**Fig. 11.24**).
- Balance on your right leg by simultaneously contracting your right quadriceps femoris to extend your front knee and your left hamstrings and left gluteus maximus (**Fig. 11.4**) to extend your left thigh. Work toward lifting the left thigh and leg so they are parallel to your mat while keeping a microbend in your right knee to protect the joint.
- Dorsiflex the left ankle, using the muscles of the anterior compartment of the leg (**Fig. 11.14**). Point your left toes down to help square off both hips, promoting internal rotation of the left thigh, using gluteus medius, gluteus minimus, tensor fasciae latae, and adductor magnus (**Fig. 11.11**).
- Keep your forearms extended and hands out in front of you or extend your arms with latissimus dorsi to press your hands together in front of your sternum.
- Use your erector spinae and the intrinsic musculature of your back to extend the vertebral column, creating a straight line from your left calcaneus to the phalanges of both hands if you extend your forearms in front of you.
- Contract your abdominals to stabilize your core and ensure that your pelvic bones are level.
- On an exhalation, release into Forward Fold (see chapter 3, forward folds) by lowering your left foot to meet your right at the top of your mat. Repeat this sequence on the other side.

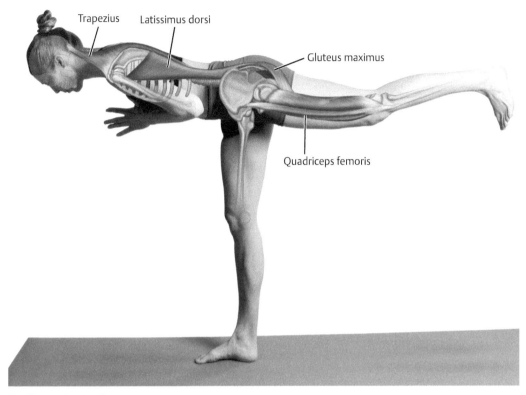

Trapezius

Latissimus dorsi

Gluteus maximus

Quadriceps femoris

Final Pose: **Warrior III**

Eagle Pose
(Garudasana)

Summary of the Pose

Named after Garuda, King of the Birds, this pose strengthens the legs, gluteal muscles, and core while also compressing every major joint in the body.

Modifications: If you are experiencing any shoulder pain, opt for a bear hug (palms to opposite shoulders) rather than the full eagle bind.

Guided Narrative

Transition 1: **One-Legged Mountain**

- From anatomical position, press your palms together anterior to your sternum and feel trapezius (**Fig. 10.7**) depress and retract your scapulae. Shift weight into the left leg and flex at your right hip to lift the right leg off the floor.
- Continue to engage your hip flexors, including iliacus and psoas major (**Fig 11.1**) to bring your right knee to the same height as your right hip. Notice that the left hip remains neutral.
- Ensure that your anterior superior iliac spines are both level and pointed forward.
- Dorsiflex the right foot through the innervation of the deep fibular nerve targeting the muscles of the anterior leg (**Fig. 11.14**).
- Lengthen through your vertebral column on your inhalations and engage your abdominal muscles (**Fig 9.5**) to help maintain balance on your exhalations.

●●

Transition 2: **Eagle Prep 1**

- With your left foot planted, flex your left knee by contracting your hamstrings (**Fig. 11.4**) and then flex both hips using sartorius and rectus femoris (**Fig. 11.1**) to bring your coccyx down closer toward the mat.
- Begin to cross your lifted right thigh over your left thigh. Option to kick stand your right toes to the earth, a block, or wrap your right toes behind the left calf.
- Your adductors (**Fig. 11.5**) are working bilaterally to squeeze your thighs together.
- Bring both knees toward the midline, noting that gracilis is contracting to maintain the internal rotation of the left tibia.

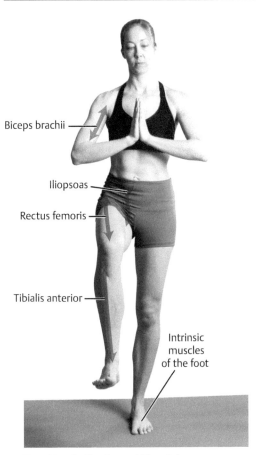

Biceps brachii

Iliopsoas

Rectus femoris

Tibialis anterior

Intrinsic muscles of the foot

Transition 1: One-Legged Mountain

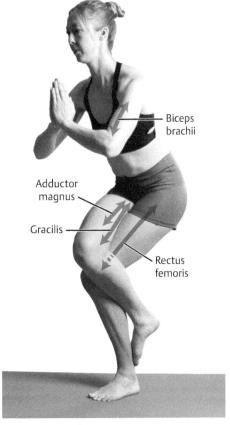

Biceps brachii

Adductor magnus

Gracilis

Rectus femoris

Transition 2: Eagle Prep 1

Transition 3: **Eagle Prep 2**

- Once you feel stable in your eagle legs, use the acromial part of deltoid and supraspinatus (**Fig. 10.2**) to abduct your arms and latissimus dorsi to extend your arms into a T-shape.
- The posterior fibers of deltoid (**Fig. 10.3**) are also aiding in this shoulder extension.
- Appreciate that the right and left triceps brachii and anconeus (**Fig. 10.11**) extend both elbows.
- Continue to adduct your inner thighs closer together using your adductors in your medial compartment.
- On your inhalations, lengthen through your vertebral column from your sacrum through your calvaria, and on your exhalations flex your hips sinking deeper into the pose.

• •

Final Pose: **Eagle Pose**

- From eagle prep 2, adduct your arms and flex both elbows by contracting biceps brachii and brachialis (**Fig. 10.10**) to swing your right elbow underneath your left. Option to keep the dorsal surface of your hands touching, or wrap your wrists and touch your palms together for a double bind.
- Notice that in the bind, both forearms are pronated by the action of pronator teres and pronator quadratus (**Fig. 10.12**) supplied by the median nerve.
- Draw your elbows up to the same height as your shoulders and extend the vertebral column to stack your shoulders over your hips.
- Continue to adduct and internally rotate your thighs. Note that your gluteus medius and minimus (**Fig. 11.4**) are working to maintain hip flexion in this pose.
- On an exhalation, unwind your arms and legs allowing blood to flow back to the muscles surrounding the joints. Repeat on the other side with your left leg wrapped on top of right, and your left elbow wrapped under right.

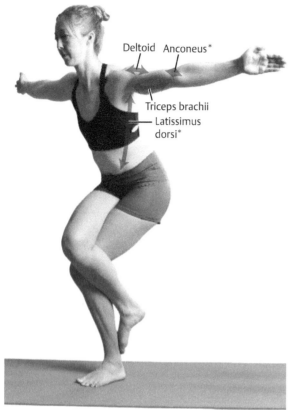

Deltoid   Anconeus*

Triceps brachii

Latissimus
dorsi*

Transition 3: **Eagle Prep 2**

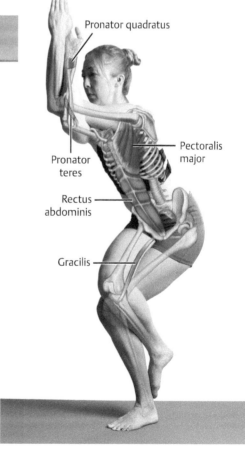

Pronator quadratus

Pectoralis
major

Pronator
teres

Rectus
abdominis

Gracilis

Final Pose: **Eagle Pose**

Half Moon II
(Ardha Chandrasana II)

Summary of the Pose

Named after the balancing energies of the sun and moon, this pose strengthens the abdomen, thighs, and vertebral column while stretching the groin/inner thigh, hamstrings, and chest. It promotes the dual sensations of both grounding and lifting in the body.

Modifications: Use a block under the bottom hand for extra support to lengthen both sides of the torso evenly. You can also practice this pose with your back leaning against a wall.

Guided Narrative

Transition 1: **Warrior II**

- Begin in anatomical position. Use gluteus medius and gluteus minimus (**Fig. 11.4**) to abduct your left hip and step your feet wide into Warrior II (see chapter 1, standing poses). Align the calcaneus of your right foot with the middle of the arch of the left foot.
- Notice that your right hamstrings (**Fig. 11.4**) are flexing your front knee and your left quadriceps femoris extends the back knee.
- Feel supraspinatus and deltoid (**Fig. 10.2**) abduct your arms out to the sides.
- Extend your forearms, wrists, and digits so they are parallel to the floor with palms facing down and align your shoulder joints superior to the hip joints.
- Find your *drishti* (gaze) past your right third distal phalanx by contracting your left sternocleidomastoid and right splenius capitis (**Fig. 9.1**).

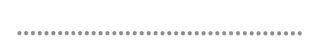

Transition 2: **Extended Side Angle**

- Flex your torso laterally to the right by ipsilaterally contracting your right internal and external obliques, erector spinae, and quadratus lumborum (**Fig. 9.6**).
- Place your right palm to the ground or to a block medial to your right foot. Alternatively, place your right forearm on your thigh.
- Feel deltoid (**Fig. 10.3**) abduct your left arm at the shoulder, inhaling your hand to the ceiling, extending your fingers at the interphalangeal joints.
- Turn your gaze up to your left hand using your right sternocleidomastoid and left splenius capitis.
- Lengthen the crown of your head toward the front of the room during your inhalations and twist your torso to the ceiling on your exhalations, moving to stack your left shoulder superior to your right shoulder.

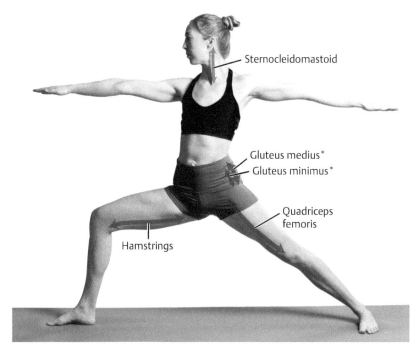

Sternocleidomastoid

Gluteus medius*
Gluteus minimus*

Quadriceps
femoris

Hamstrings

Transition 1: Warrior II

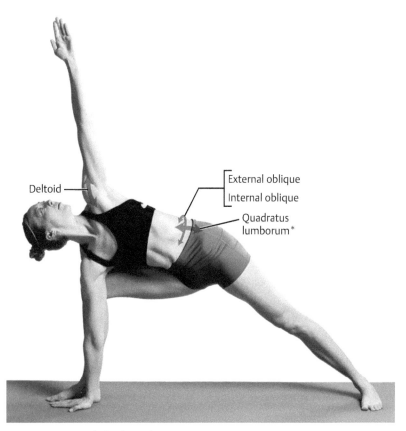

Deltoid

External oblique
Internal oblique

Quadratus
lumborum*

Transition 2: Extended Side Angle

Final Pose: **Half Moon**

- Bring your right fingertips to the mat or to a block about six inches in front of your right foot. Begin to abduct your left leg to lift it off the mat, contracting tensor fascia latae, and continuing to dorsiflex the left foot. Imagine you are kicking the back wall, using your left tibialis anterior along with other dorsiflexors of the left foot (**Fig. 11.14**).
- Observe quadriceps femoris extending your knees in both the standing and the lifted leg.
- As you reach for the mat or a block, your right psoas major (**Fig. 11.1**) supplied by L1–L3 spinal nerves and iliacus supplied by the femoral nerve (L2–L4) are working to flex at the hip.
- Gaze can be down to your mat or option to look up toward your left fingertips to challenge your balance if comfortable.
- On an exhalation, slowly step the left foot to the back of your mat and bring your torso upright returning to Warrior II. Step your feet together at the top of your mat and repeat this sequence on the other side.

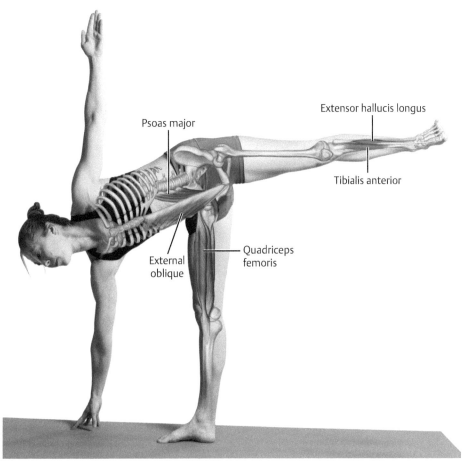

Extensor hallucis longus

Psoas major

Tibialis anterior

Quadriceps femoris

External oblique

Final Pose: **Half Moon**

King Dancer
(Natarajasana)

Summary of the Pose

This sequence of poses works toward a deep backbend, strengthening the extensor muscles of the vertebral column and stretching the muscles across the thorax and shoulders. The extensors of the standing leg and intrinsic muscles of the foot strongly contract to maintain balance and improve proprioception.

Modifications: Bring the palm of your free hand to a wall or chair for stability.

Guided Narrative

Transition 1: **Dancer Prep 1**

- Begin in anatomical position. Contract your left hamstrings to flex the left leg and reach for the medial side of your left foot with your left hand, externally rotating your left shoulder using teres minor and infraspinatus (**Fig. 10.2**).
- Keep both thighs and knees together by contracting adductor magnus (**Fig. 11.1**).
- Note that your tibial nerve will allow your left foot to plantarflex by contracting the muscles of the posterior compartment of your left leg (**Fig. 11.16**).
- Inhale your right hand to the ceiling by flexing your right shoulder, using the clavicular part of deltoid and coracobrachialis (**Fig. 10.5**).

● ●

Transition 2: **Dancer**

- Begin to hinge forward, kicking your left foot into your left hand and extending your right fingertips out in front of you.
- To prevent the left knee from drifting laterally, use gluteus medius, gluteus minimus, and tensor fasciae latae (**Fig. 11.1**) to internally rotate the left thigh at the hip.
- Continue to plantarflex your left foot visualizing the actions of soleus and gastrocnemius. Find balance by gripping the mat with all four corners of your right foot to engage the intrinsic muscles of the foot.
- Observe your left iliacus, psoas major, and rectus femoris (**Fig. 11.1**) lengthen as you kick your left leg back.
- Feel a stretch across your left pectoralis major and the clavicular part of your left deltoid.
- Work to square your chest to the mat by moving your left scapula laterally and anteriorly. All three parts of serratus anterior (**Fig. 10.6**) help with this action.

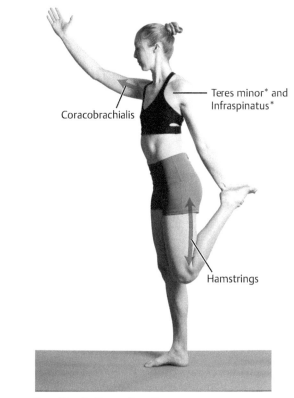

Coracobrachialis

Teres minor* and
Infraspinatus*

Hamstrings

Transition 1: **Dancer Prep 1**

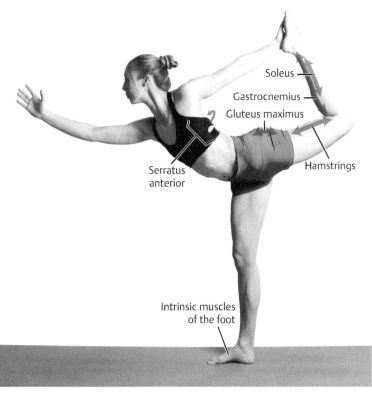

Soleus

Gastrocnemius

Gluteus maximus

Hamstrings

Serratus
anterior

Intrinsic muscles
of the foot

Transition 2: **Dancer**

Final Pose: **King Dancer (with a strap)**

- To work into a deeper expression of this pose, wrap a strap around the arch of your left foot.
- While holding the strap in one hand, use both deltoid muscles to abduct your shoulders and extend your arms overhead.
- Grab the strap with both hands superior and posterior to your head and then utilize brachialis (**Fig. 10.10**) in both arms to flex the elbows.
- Begin to kick your left foot into the strap as you hinge your torso forward.
- On an inhalation, feel the muscles of your back extend your vertebral column and use soleus and gastrocnemius to strongly plantarflex your left foot.
- On an exhalation, lift your torso back up as you remove your left foot from the strap and bring your left foot back to the mat. Repeat this sequence on the other side.

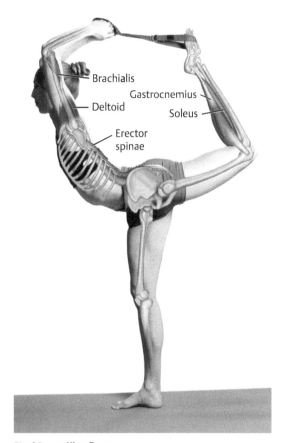

Brachialis

Deltoid

Erector spinae

Gastrocnemius

Soleus

Final Pose: **King Dancer**

3 Forward Folds

Standing Forward Fold and Gorilla
(Uttanasana and Padahastasana)

Summary of the Pose

Forward folds stretch the calves, hamstrings, back, and neck and are said to help calm the mind.

Modifications: If your hamstrings are tight, bend your knees generously in the forward fold. Option to bring a block underneath your palms.

Guided Narrative

Transition 1: **Forward Fold**

- From anatomical position, contract your abdominals to flex your vertebral column and fold forward bringing your chest close to your thighs. Option to keep your halluces touching or separate your feet hips-width apart.
- Relax your head and neck and draw your head closer to your thighs gazing between your legs. Only fold as deep as is comfortable.
- Lift your patellae proximally by contracting quadriceps femoris (**Fig. 11.1**) to feel a deep stretch across your hamstrings (**Fig. 11.4**).
- In this fold, your vertebral column is in mild flexion and your spinal extensors (**Fig. 8.2**) are lengthening.
- As you place your hands down on the mat or a block, notice that your triceps brachii (**Fig. 10.11**) work to extend the elbow joints.

• •

Transition 2: **Halfway Lift**

- From Forward Fold, inhale and feel erector spinae extend your vertebral column into a halfway lift. Press your fingertips into the mat or bring your palms to your tibias.
- Activate your quadriceps femoris muscles to lift your patellae proximally.
- Through the innervation of the superior gluteal nerve, use gluteus medius, gluteus minimus, and tensor fascia latae (**Table 11.4**) to keep both thighs internally rotated in this pose.
- Create one long line from your coccyx through your hip and shoulder joints, and out the crown of your head. Notice that trapezius (**Fig. 8.1**) helps to draw both scapulae medially and down your back.
- Use splenius capitis to extend your neck and bring your gaze (*drishti*) a few inches in front of you.
- Release the lift on an exhalation and use your abdominals to flex back into a forward fold.

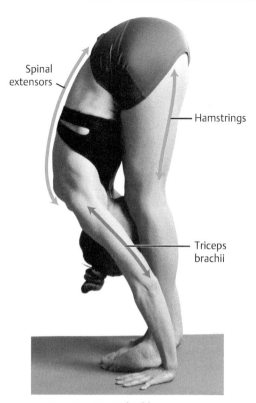

Spinal extensors

Hamstrings

Triceps brachii

Transition 1: **Forward Fold**

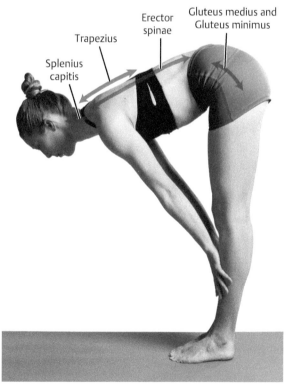

Trapezius

Erector spinae

Gluteus medius and Gluteus minimus

Splenius capitis

Transition 2: **Halfway Lift**

Final Pose: **Gorilla**

- Start to walk your hands in front of your feet and press the dorsum of your hands onto the mat with your fingers facing your toes. Begin with your knees flexed then slowly begin to extend your knees as is comfortable.
- Slide your hands under the plantar surface of your feet until your toes touch your flexor retinacula.
- Use biceps brachii, brachialis, and brachioradialis (**Fig. 10.12**) to flex your forearms, pointing the elbows laterally to help draw your chest closer to your thighs.
- Exhale and bring more weight into the metatarsal heads of both feet.
- Press your toes into your wrists for a light massage on the carpal tunnel and the flexor tendons of your forearm's anterior compartment.
- Release your hands and slowly rise up through each region of your vertebral column to return to anatomical position.

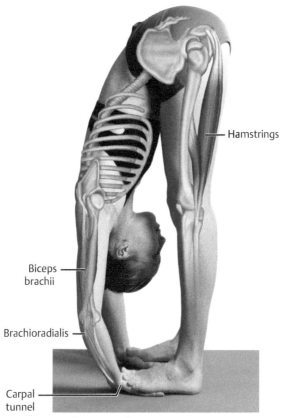

Hamstrings

Biceps
brachii

Brachioradialis

Carpal
tunnel

Final Pose: **Gorilla**

Pyramid
(Parsvottanasana)

Summary of the Pose

This pose stretches the back, shoulders, and hamstrings while compressing the thyroid gland.

Modifications: Bring blocks underneath both palms before folding forward. Option to flex deeply through your knees if you experience back or hamstring pain.

Guided Narrative

Transition 1: **Low Lunge**

- From anatomical position, step your left foot toward the back of your mat. Use your right hamstrings to flex your knee and ensure it tracks directly above your right ankle.
- Place both palms on either side of your right foot and note that the clavicular part of deltoid (**Fig. 10.1**) aids in flexion of the shoulder.
- Contract your abdominals (**Fig. 9.5**) to flex your vertebral column and draw your umbilicus up and in, away from your right thigh.
- Bilaterally contract splenius capitis and longissimus capitis (**Fig. 8.3**) to slightly extend your head at the neck to gaze a few inches in front of your mat. Recall that these deep back muscles are innervated by dorsal rami.
- As you push into the ground, feel serratus anterior (**Fig. 10.6**) protract your scapulae and your hamstrings and gluteus maximus (**Fig. 11.4**) extend your left thigh.

• •

Transition 2: **Pyramid Prep**

- Shorten your stance by stepping your left foot closer to the top of your mat while keeping your back foot at a 45-degree angle. Align the calcaneus of your front foot with the calcaneus of your back foot.
- Use quadriceps femoris, supplied by the femoral nerve, to extend both knees.
- Ground down through both heels and feel the stretch in the posterior compartment of your legs, including gastrocnemius and soleus (**Fig. 11.16**).
- Use your triceps brachii (**Fig. 10.11**) to extend both elbows and inhale up onto your fingertips, lengthening the crown of your head anteriorly to the front of the room. If you are unable to reach the mat, place a block under each palm.
- Use the descending fibers of trapezius to depress both scapulae and draw your shoulders away from your ears.
- Maintain this pose with a flat back for a couple rounds of breath.

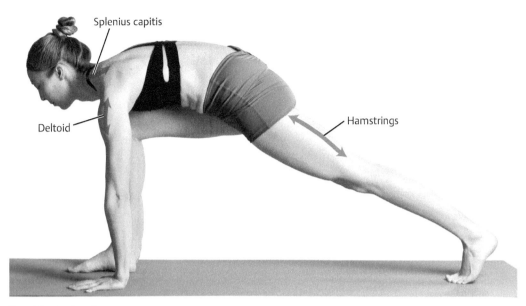

Splenius capitis

Deltoid

Hamstrings

Transition 2: **Low Lunge**

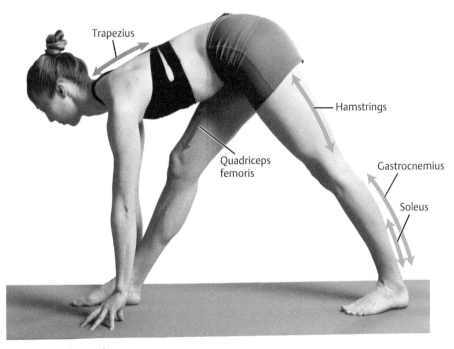

Trapezius

Hamstrings

Quadriceps femoris

Gastrocnemius

Soleus

Transition 2: **Pyramid Prep**

Final Pose: **Pyramid**

- On an exhalation, begin to flex at your hips and contract rectus abdominis to bow your torso over your front right leg. Depending on what feels comfortable, rest your forehead on your knee or draw your mandible toward your shin.
- Maintain extension in both knee joints and feel the stretch in your hamstrings.
- Contract brachialis and brachioradialis (**Fig. 10.12**) to flex your elbows, helping to bring your chest closer to your right thigh.
- Note that your gluteus medius and minimus muscles help to flex and internally rotate both hips.
- To exit the pose, step your left foot to meet your right in Standing Forward Fold. Exhale and step your right foot back to a low lunge and repeat this sequence on the other side.

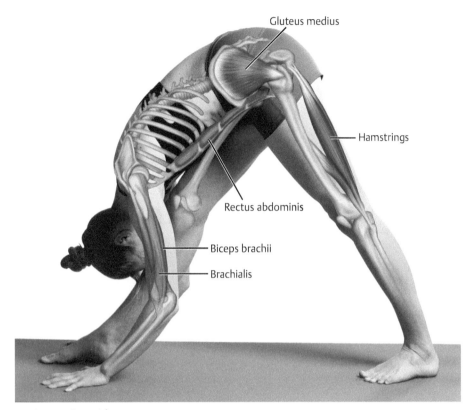

Gluteus medius

Hamstrings

Rectus abdominis

Biceps brachii

Brachialis

Final Pose: **Pyramid**

Seated Head to Knee
(Janu Sirsasna)

Summary of the Pose

This pose helps calm the mind, stretches the muscles of the lower back and the hamstrings. It is believed to relieve headaches, stress, and insomnia.

Modifications: Sit up on a blanket to promote an anterior pelvic tilt. Place a block under your flexed knee for additional support.

Guided Narrative

Transition 1: **Staff Pose**

- From a seated position, bring both legs out in front of you, using quadriceps femoris (**Fig. 11.12**) to extend both knees.
- Press your hands into the mat on either side of your pelvis while triceps brachii (**Fig. 10.11**) extends both elbows.
- Contract tibialis anterior (**Fig. 11.14**) to dorsiflex both feet and point your toes up to the ceiling, recalling that this muscle is innervated by the deep fibular nerve.
- Ground down through your ischial tuberosities and use erector spinae (**Fig. 8.3**) to extend and lengthen your trunk and neck.

• •

Transition 2: **Seated Head to Knee Prep**

- Use your left hamstrings (**Fig. 11.4**) to flex your left knee and bring the sole of the left foot to the medial right thigh. Keep the right leg extended.
- Your left obturator internus and obturator externus (**Fig. 11.5**) are working to externally rotate your hip.
- Note that pectineus and adductor magnus (**Fig. 11.1**) help to adduct your right hip and internal rotation is aided by adductor magnus, gluteus medius, and gluteus minimus.
- Continue to use the muscles of the anterior compartment of your legs to dorsiflex both feet.
- While maintaining axial extension, begin to flex your vertebral column forward over your extended right leg by contracting rectus abdominis (**Fig. 9.7**). Bring a strap around your right foot to assist in folding deeper.

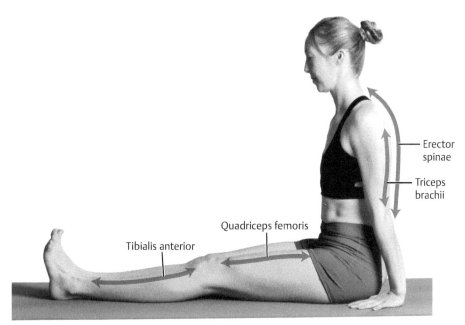

Erector spinae

Triceps brachii

Quadriceps femoris

Tibialis anterior

Transition 1: **Staff Pose**

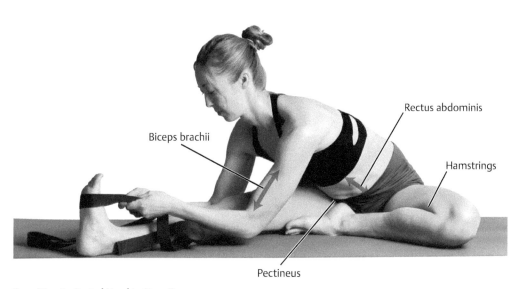

Rectus abdominis

Biceps brachii

Hamstrings

Pectineus

Transition 2: **Seated Head to Knee Prep**

Final Pose: **Seated Head to Knee**

- On an inhalation, extend your vertebral column to sit back up and use your deltoids to abduct both arms overhead, externally rotating your shoulders.
- Use your abdominal obliques to slightly rotate your torso so that you directly face your extended right leg.
- On an exhalation, flex at your hips to lower your torso toward your right leg. Place your hands wherever is accessible: feet, ankles, or shins. If comfortable, draw your forehead to your right knee.
- As you fold, feel the stretch in your low back, including in your left quadratus lumborum (**Fig. 8.2**).
- Continue to externally rotate and flex the left hip, utilizing sartorius (**Table 11.5**) supplied by the femoral nerve.
- To exit this pose, extend your spine to return to a seated position by contracting erector spinae. Repeat this sequence on the other side with your right knee flexed and your left knee extended.

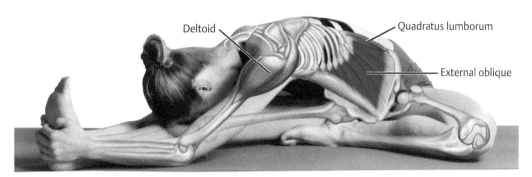

Deltoid

Quadratus lumborum

External oblique

Final Pose: **Seated Head to Knee**

Bound Angle
(Baddha Konasana)

Summary of the Pose

Sometimes referred to as Butterfly or Cobbler's Pose, this seated forward bend simultaneously stretches the hips and back.

Modifications: If your hips are tight, sit on a blanket to promote an anterior pelvic tilt which will allow you to fold deeper in this pose. Rest your forehead or forearms onto a block when folding forward for more support.

Guided Narrative

Transition 1: **Staff Pose**

- From a seated position, extend both legs out in front of you, using quadriceps femoris (**Fig. 11.12**) to extend both knees.
- Press your hands into the mat on either side of your pelvis while triceps brachii (**Fig. 10.11**) extends both the elbows.
- Contract tibialis anterior (**Fig. 11.14**) to dorsiflex both feet and point your toes up to the ceiling.
- Ground down through your ischial tuberosities and use your erector spinae (**Fig. 8.3**) to extend and lengthen your spine and neck.

● ●

Transition 2: **Bound Angle Prep**

- Contract sartorius and your hamstrings (**Fig. 11.13**) to flex both knees, drawing the plantar surfaces of your feet to touch.
- Interlace your fingers around your halluces then depress and retract your scapulae using trapezius and your rhomboids (**Fig. 8.1**).
- Feel your thighs externally rotating from the action of the lateral rotators of the hip: piriformis, superior gemellus, and inferior gemellus (**Fig. 11.4**).
- Work toward gradually moving your thighs toward the floor and your patellae laterally; place a block under each knee for additional support if needed.
- Continue to extend through your spine from your sacrum to your external occipital protuberance and align your shoulders over your hips.

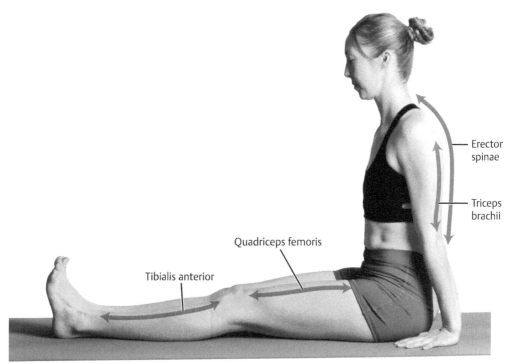

Erector
spinae

Triceps
brachii

Quadriceps femoris

Tibialis anterior

Transition 1: **Staff Pose**

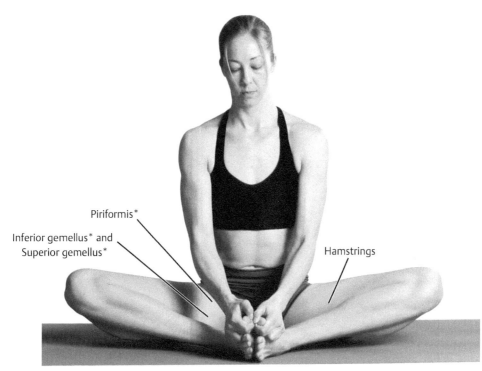

Piriformis*

Inferior gemellus* and
Superior gemellus*

Hamstrings

Transition 2: **Bound Angle Prep**

Final Pose: **Bound Angle**

- From Bound Angle Prep, exhale and flex your vertebral column forward over your legs.
- Depress and retract your scapulae using trapezius and your rhomboids.
- Continue to engage erector spinae (iliocostalis, longissimus, and spinalis) to lengthen the vertebral column and avoid rounding your neck and back.
- Feel the stretch across the anterior part of your deltoid, appreciating the fact that it is innervated by the axillary nerve.
- Stay in this fold for three to four rounds of breath then extend through the vertebral column to return to an upright position.

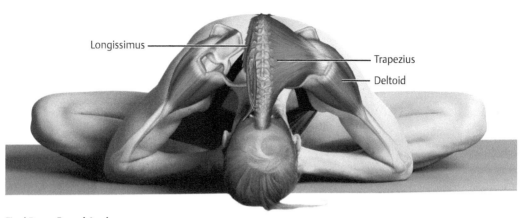

Longissimus

Trapezius

Deltoid

Final Pose: **Bound Angle**

King Pigeon
(Eka Pada Rajakapotasana)

Summary of the Pose

This pose stretches the gluteals of the flexed front leg and the hip flexors of the extended back leg. As an intense hip opener, it is said to promote introspection.

Modifications: Use a block or folded blanket under the thigh of the flexed leg to help level your hips. When folded forward, rest your forehead on the mat, forearms, a block, or a blanket for additional support. If you experience knee pain in this pose take the "supine pigeon" variation: lay on your back with both feet on the mat, keep your left knee flexed while you cross your right ankle over your left thigh, with an option to draw your left knee toward your chest.

Guided Narrative

Transition 1: **Three-Legged Down Dog**

- From Downward Facing Dog, use gluteus maximus and the hamstrings (**Fig. 11.4**) to extend your right thigh at the hip, lifting your right leg into the air.
- Push your hands into the ground and feel serratus anterior protracting your scapulae and trapezius (**Fig. 8.1**) depressing your scapulae, creating space between your ears and shoulders.
- With quadriceps femoris (**Fig. 11.12**) extending your knees, feel a stretch along the muscles of the posterior compartment of your grounded left leg.
- Use tibialis anterior (**Fig. 11.14**) to dorsiflex your right foot and angle your toes toward the ground to help internally rotate your right hip.

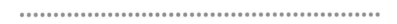

Transition 2: **Low Lunge**

- Using your hip flexors, bring your right knee toward your nose and slowly contract quadriceps femoris to extend your right leg, placing the plantar surface of the right foot to the ground between the palms.
- Align the patella of your right knee superior to your ankle.
- Contract your abdominals (**Fig. 9.5**) to flex your vertebral column and draw your umbilicus up and in, away from your right thigh.
- Bilaterally contract trapezius, splenius capitis, and longissimus capitis (**Fig. 8.3**) to slightly extend your head at the neck to gaze a few inches in front of your mat.
- As you push into the ground, feel serratus anterior (**Fig. 10.6**) protract your scapulae and notice that your hamstrings and gluteus maximus are working to extend your left thigh at the hip.

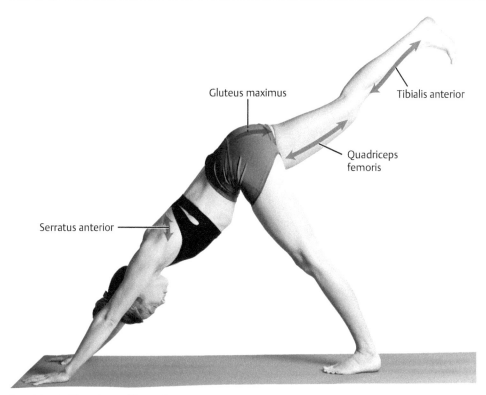

Gluteus maximus

Tibialis anterior

Quadriceps femoris

Serratus anterior

Transition 1: **Three-Legged Down Dog**

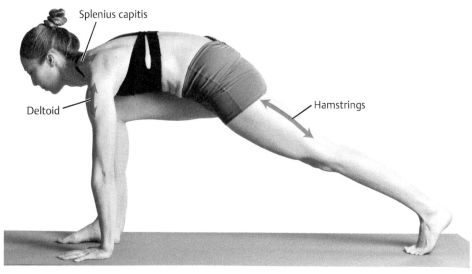

Splenius capitis

Deltoid

Hamstrings

Transition 2: **Low Lunge**

Transition 3: **Pigeon Prep**

- Externally rotate your right thigh using sartorius and the lateral rotators of the hip (**Fig. 11.5**). Gently place the lateral compartment of your right leg to the floor in front of you.
- Align your anterior superior iliac spines with the front of the mat to square the hips and keep your sacrum level. Utilize erector spinae (**Fig. 8.3**) to extend your vertebral column.
- Feel the stretch across the muscles of your right gluteal region and left hip flexors.
- Option to "put your pigeon to sleep," first flex your torso to fold over your front leg, and then bilaterally contract the clavicular part of deltoid and coracobrachialis to flex your arms out in front of you along the ground.

• •

Final Pose: **King Pigeon Pose (with strap)**

- If you are flexed forward, slowly begin to engage erector spinae to extend your vertebral column lifting your torso upright.
- Contract your left hamstrings to flex the leg, then use latissimus dorsi and the spinal part of deltoid (**Fig. 10.2**) to extend your left arm toward the back of your mat. Wrap your fingers around your left medial malleolus and draw your foot closer to your body.
- Stay with your hand to the medial malleolus, or take one of several options to continue stretching in this pose: (1) Loop a strap around the left foot and hold the strap with one or both hands (as seen in the image on next page); (2) Guide your foot into your left cubital fossa and interlace your fingers; or (3) Wrap both hands around your foot and draw the foot toward the crown of your head.
- Continue to maintain level alignment of your hips by pointing your anterior superior iliac spines toward the front of your mat and contract the muscles of your pelvic floor to support you in this pose. Engagement of the pelvic floor is known as *mula bandha*, or root lock, in some yoga philosophies.
- Exhale and slowly release the left foot returning back to the previous pose.
- Move back to Three-Legged Down Dog and circumduct your right thigh to create some gentle hip circles as a counter-movement before repeating this sequence on the other side.

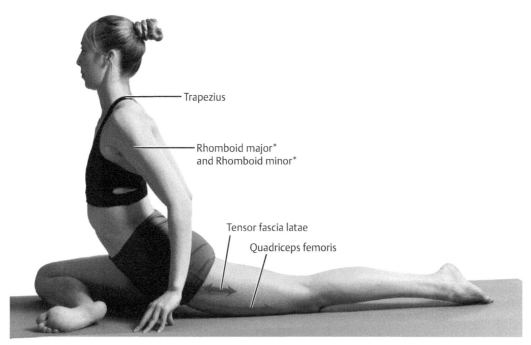

Trapezius

Rhomboid major*
and Rhomboid minor*

Tensor fascia latae

Quadriceps femoris

Transition 1: **Pigeon Prep**

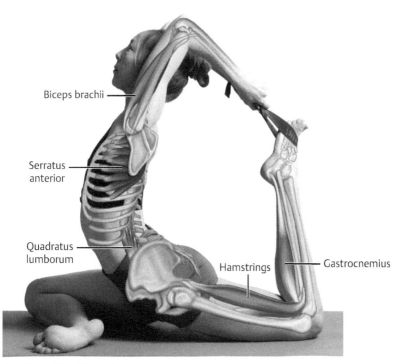

Biceps brachii

Serratus
anterior

Quadratus
lumborum

Hamstrings

Gastrocnemius

Final Pose: **King Pigeon Pose**

4 Backbends

Cobra and Locust
(Bhujangasana and Salabhasana)

Summary of the Pose

This backbend strengthens the back muscles and stretches muscles of the chest and upper abdomen.

Modifications: There are many hand variations available in this pose. You have the option of interlocking your fingers behind your back for more of a shoulder opener. You can also bring your fingertips to rest at the back of your head and lift the elbows to the ceiling.

Guided Narrative

Transition 1: **Cobra Prep**

- From Plank (see chapter 4, Upward Facing Dog, transition 1) contract biceps brachii, coracobrachialis, and brachialis (all receiving their innervation from the musculocutaneous nerve) to flex your forearms and lower down onto your abdomen. Point your elbows posteriorly toward the back of the mat and keep them close to your rib cage while lowering down. Walk your hands directly under the shoulder joints.
- On an inhalation, engage erector spinae (**Fig. 8.2**) to extend your cervical and upper thoracic vertebrae, lifting your head and chest off of the mat.
- Place little to no weight in your hands or lift your hands off of the mat. Keep your gaze down toward the mat to protect your neck. Use rhomboid major and rhomboid minor (**Fig. 10.8**) to draw your scapulae medially.
- Engage quadriceps femoris (**Fig. 11.1**) to fully extend your legs, lifting your chest a little higher. Plantarflex your feet with the help of gastrocnemius and soleus to press the dorsum of your feet into the mat.
- Hold this pose for a couple rounds of breath. On an exhalation, lower back down onto your chest.

• •

Transition 2: **Cobra**

- From prone, press into your palms and lift your chest higher using triceps brachii (**Fig. 10.11**) to extend your elbows.
- Your intrinsic back muscles are still working to extend the spine, specifically in the lumbar and thoracic regions.
- Retract and depress your scapulae. Keep your elbows close to your ribcage.
- Depending on the height of your chest, you may feel a stretch in your psoas major and rectus abdominis (**Fig. 9.7**).
- Stay active through the thighs and legs, observing adductor magnus extending, adducting, and internally rotating your hips.
- Notice that your forearms are pronated in this pose, so both pronator quadratus and pronator teres are utilized (**Fig. 10.12**).
- On an exhalation, lower back down to your chest and torso.

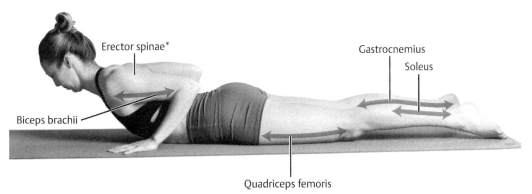

Erector spinae*

Gastrocnemius

Soleus

Biceps brachii

Quadriceps femoris

Transition 1: **Cobra Prep**

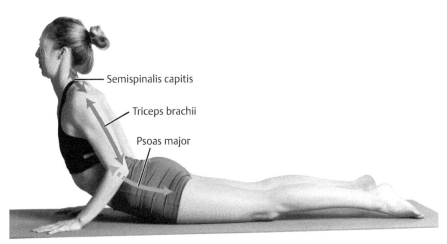

Semispinalis capitis

Triceps brachii

Psoas major

Transition 2: **Cobra**

Final Pose: **Locust**

- Lie prone on your mat and extend your arms along your sides. Bring your forehead to the mat.
- On your next inhalation, engage your spinal extensors to lift through your chest while simultaneously lifting your arms, legs, and feet off of the mat. If comfortable, utilize triceps brachii to extend both elbows and reach your fingertips toward your calcanei.
- Anchor your body to the mat using your lower abdominals and pelvis in this variation.
- Use serratus anterior (**Fig. 10.6**) to upwardly rotate your scapulae and trapezius to retract and depress your scapulae.
- Appreciate that your hamstrings and gluteus maximus are maintaining the extension of both hips.
- Utilize the muscles in the posterior compartment of your legs, including gastrocnemius and soleus (**Fig. 11.16**), to plantarflex both feet toward the back of your mat.
- Hold this pose for several rounds of breath and release back down to the mat on an exhalation.

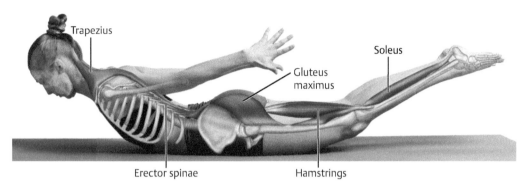

Trapezius

Soleus

Gluteus
maximus

Erector spinae

Hamstrings

Final Pose: **Locust**

Upward Facing Dog
(Urdhva Mukha Svanasana)

Summary of the Pose

This backbend is an important pose in *vinyasa* styles of yoga and stretches the chest and abdomen while strengthening the wrists, arms, and shoulders.

Modifications: If you experience low back pain, modify this pose with Cobra Prep (refer to the previous pose sequence).

Guided Narrative

Transition 1: **Plank**

- From Table Top (see chapter 4, Camel, transition 1), step both feet back utilizing your hamstrings (**Fig. 11.4**) to extend both hips and then quadriceps femoris (**Fig. 11.1**) to extend both knees pressing your toes into the mat behind you.
- Dorsiflex through your ankles using the muscles of the anterior compartment of your leg, including tibialis anterior, extensor digitorum longus, and extensor hallucis longus.
- Stack your shoulders superior to your wrists and strongly press through your palms to protract your scapulae, utilizing the long thoracic nerve to engage serratus anterior (**Fig. 10.6**).
- Bilaterally contract splenius to look slightly forward maintaining the length in your neck.
- Muscles of the rotator cuff (**Fig. 10.4**) are helping to stabilize your shoulder joints here.
- Begin to strengthen your core finding a posterior pelvic tilt by drawing your pubis towards the top of your mat, engaging your rectus abdominis and transversus abdominis muscles (**Fig. 9.5**).

• •

Transition 2: **Four-Limbed Staff**

- While maintaining equal weight distribution across your palms, inhale and hinge forward coming to the tops of your toes. Exhale and use biceps brachii and brachialis to lower halfway, keeping your elbows close to your ribcage and flexed at a 90-degree angle or less.
- Notice that pectoralis major is assisting in the adduction of both humeri.
- Continue to engage rectus abdominis to further strengthen your core, your hamstrings to extend both hips, and quadriceps femoris to extend both knees.
- Stay active through the thighs, observing adductor magnus (**Fig. 11.3**) adducting and internally rotating your hips.
- If you feel unstable here, lower down to your patellae.

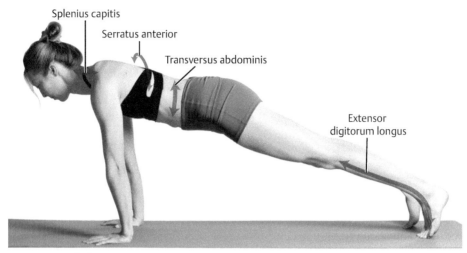

Splenius capitis

Serratus anterior

Transversus abdominis

Extensor
digitorum longus

Transition 1: **Plank**

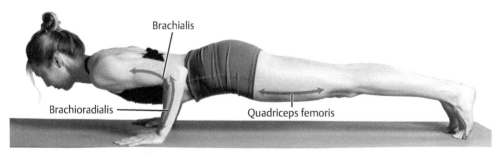

Brachialis

Brachioradialis

Quadriceps femoris

Transition 2: **Four-Limbed Staff**

Final Pose: **Upward Facing Dog**

- Shift forward and plantarflex your feet to place the dorsal surface to the mat. Notice this movement contracts the muscles of the posterior compartment (**Fig. 11.16**) and lateral compartment of the legs, including fibularis longus and brevis (**Fig. 11.15**).
- Acknowledge your radial nerves innervating triceps brachii as you press into your palms to extend your elbows. Slightly arch backward through your thoracic spine, engaging your spinal extensor muscles, such as multifidus (**Fig. 8.2**). If comfortable, further extend the cervical spine and gaze upward.
- Keep your thighs lifted off the mat by engaging quadriceps femoris. Focus on the adduction and internal rotation of your hips by adductor magnus.
- Depress your scapulae with the ascending (lower) fibers of trapezius.
- Avoid rounding forward in your upper body. Use infraspinatus and teres minor (**Fig. 10.2**) to externally rotate your shoulders, and the middle fibers of trapezius and the rhomboids to retract your scapulae, further stretching the chest.
- On an exhalation, release from this pose by lifting your hips, dorsiflexing your ankles to return the plantar surface of your toes to the mat, and press back to Downward Facing Dog (see chapter 5, arm balances).

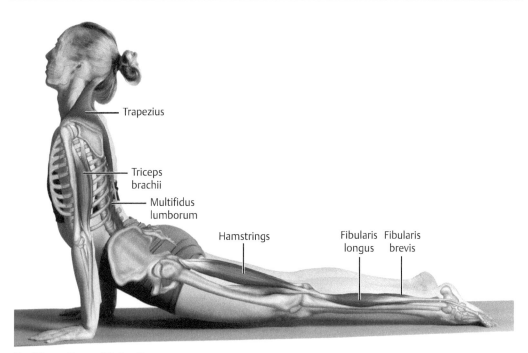

Trapezius

Triceps
brachii

Multifidus
lumborum

Hamstrings

Fibularis
longus

Fibularis
brevis

Final Pose: **Upward Facing Dog**

Camel
(Ustrasana)

Summary of the Pose

This backbend is an invigorating heart opener. It helps to strengthen the spinal extensors while stretching the ventral side of the body.

Modifications: Keep the feet dorsiflexed and toes tucked under (seen in transition 3) if the final pose is uncomfortable. Place blocks on the outside of the ankles to support you in the final transitions of this backbend.

Guided Narrative

Transition 1: **Table Top**

- From a seated position, plant your palms into the mat and extend your legs behind you, stacking your shoulders superior to your wrists and your hips over your knees.
- Use your triceps brachii (**Fig. 10.11**) to extend both elbows and your dorsal interossei of the hands (**Fig. 10.15**) to abduct and spread your fingers wide creating a firm base.
- Notice that your hamstrings (**Fig. 11.4**) are working to flex both knees.
- Look about six inches in front of you by contracting trapezius (**Fig. 10.7**) to create a neutral vertebral column.

●●

Transition 2: **Camel Prep 1**

- Keep your thighs hips-width distance apart and rise up to your knees, feeling the muscles along your spine extend your trunk.
- Internally rotate both femurs through the action of gluteus medius and gluteus minimus (**Fig. 11.9**), and use your adductors and gracilis (**Fig. 11.3**) to squeeze your inner thighs toward the midline. Option to place a block between your thighs to promote this internal rotation.
- Using brachioradialis and biceps brachii (**Fig. 10.10**), flex both elbows and rest your palms on your sacrum with your fingers pointing inferiorly using extensor digitorum (**Fig. 10.13**).
- Engage your rectus abdominis (**Fig. 9.5**) and extend through the spine to help stack your shoulders over hips and hips over knees. Retract your scapulae by contracting your rhomboids (**Fig. 10.8**), innervated by the dorsal scapular nerve.
- Option to curl your toes and bring your heels high or keep the dorsal surfaces of both feet grounded to the mat.

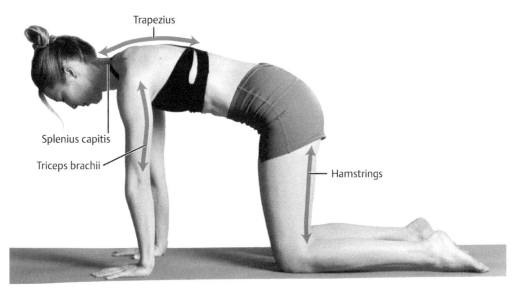

Trapezius

Splenius capitis

Triceps brachii

Hamstrings

Transition 1: **Table Top**

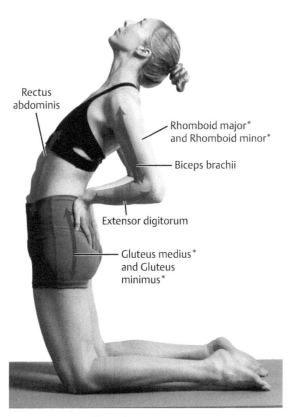

Rectus
abdominis

Rhomboid major*
and Rhomboid minor*

Biceps brachii

Extensor digitorum

Gluteus medius*
and Gluteus
minimus*

Transition 2: **Camel Prep 1**

Transition 3: **Camel Prep 2**

- On an exhalation, continue to extend through your vertebral column as you lift your chest superiorly and then posteriorly, shifting your gaze toward the ceiling. Extend only as far as is comfortable here.
- Take small sips of air in this backbend. Stay here with your palms on your sacrum or move deeper into this pose by externally rotating your right shoulder using infraspinatus (**Fig. 10.4**). Extend your right forearm with triceps brachii and reach for your right calcaneus or a block.
- Visualize the divisions of erector spinae (**Fig. 8.2**) as you extend through the spine and appreciate quadratus lumborum (**Fig. 9.6**) contracting to further extend your back.
- To challenge your balance, bring your left hand to your sternum.

• •

Final Pose: **Camel**

- Continue to dorsiflex your feet or activate the muscles of the posterior compartment of your legs (**Fig. 11.16**) to plantarflex your ankles, placing the dorsum of the feet on the mat.
- To deepen this backbend, lengthen through the vertebral column on an inhalation and lift through the chest. On an exhalation, use your left triceps brachii to extend your forearm reaching for your left calcaneus or a block.
- Continue to engage erector spinae and quadratus lumborum for spinal extension, maintain the lift in your chest, and feel your rectus abdominis engaged to support your low back.
- Your sternocleidomastoid muscles stretch and lengthen as you extend through the cervical spine.
- Stay for a few rounds of breath, taking small inhalations in this deep backbend.
- To release this pose, return to transition 2 by bringing your palms to the low back, tuck your chin, and contract your abdominals to slowly flex the vertebral column to rise.
- Take a counter pose, such as Child's Pose to fully flex the spine.

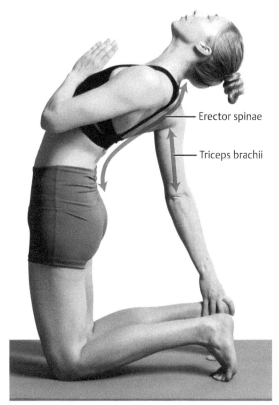

Erector spinae

Triceps brachii

Transition 3: **Camel Prep 2**

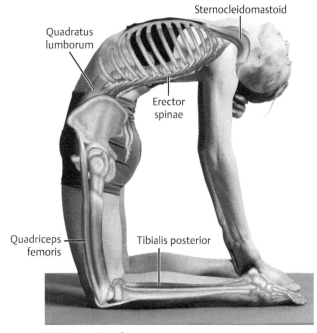

Sternocleidomastoid

Quadratus lumborum

Erector spinae

Quadriceps femoris

Tibialis posterior

Final Pose: **Camel**

Bow
(Dhanurasana)

Summary of the Pose

Named after an archer's bow, this pose stretches the front of the body while strengthening the back of the body.

Modifications: Stay in either one of the prep poses or use a strap, scarf, or belt around the ankle joints if you are unable to reach them in the full expression of this pose. If pregnant, practice Camel instead of Bow (see the previous pose sequence).

Guided Narrative

Transition 1: **Cobra Prep**

- From Plank (see chapter 4, Upward Facing Dog, transition 1), contract biceps brachii, coracobrachialis, and brachialis to flex your forearms and lower down onto your abdomen. Point your elbows straight back and keep them close to your rib cage while lowering down. Walk your hands directly under the shoulder joints.
- Inhale and engage erector spinae (**Fig. 8.2**) to extend your cervical and upper thoracic vertebrae, lifting your head and chest off of the mat.
- Place little to no weight in your hands or lift your hands off of the mat. Keep your gaze down toward the mat to protect your neck. Use rhomboid major and rhomboid minor (**Fig. 10.8**) to draw your scapulae medially.
- Engage quadriceps femoris (**Fig. 11.1**) to fully extend your legs, lifting your chest a little higher. Plantarflex your feet with the help of gastrocnemius and soleus, both innervated by the tibial nerve to press the dorsum of your feet into the mat.
- Hold this pose for a couple rounds of breath. On an exhalation, release back to the mat.

• •

Transition 2: **One-Legged Bow**

- Rest your right forearm in front of you and actively push your elbow into the ground, using serratus anterior (**Fig. 10.6**) to protract your scapula.
- Continue to extend through the vertebral column and grasp your left foot or ankle with your left hand by extending and then supinating your left forearm while your hamstrings flex your left knee.
- Feel the opposing actions of plantarflexion in your right foot and dorsiflexion in your left foot.
- On your inhalations, continue to feel the extension along your vertebral column. When you are ready to release from this pose, lower down on an exhalation and repeat this transition pose on the right side.

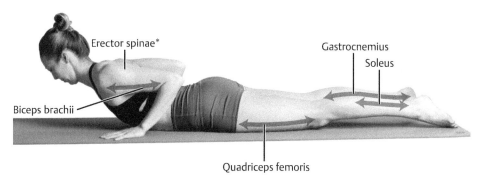

Erector spinae*

Gastrocnemius

Soleus

Biceps brachii

Quadriceps femoris

Transition 1: **Cobra Prep**

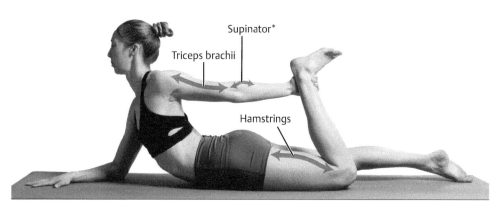

Supinator*

Triceps brachii

Hamstrings

Transition 2: **One-Legged Bow**

Final Pose: **Bow**

- On an inhalation, bilaterally contract your hamstrings to flex both knees to lift your legs off of the ground.
- Utilize latissimus dorsi and deltoid to extend through both arms and triceps brachii to extend through both forearms, reaching for your ankle joints with your fingers. Grasp your feet or ankles and maintain a neutral gaze a few inches in front of your mat.
- Engage your rhomboids and middle fibers of trapezius (**Fig. 10.7**) for scapular retraction. Feel the stretch across pectoralis major and anterior deltoid (**Fig. 10.3**) and the engagement of your abdominals to support your lower back.
- Use muscles of the anterior compartment of the leg, including extensor digitorum longus (**Fig. 11.14**) to dorsiflex both feet.
- Continue to engage erector spinae and multifidus. Slowly lower down coming out of the pose on an exhalation. Keep your knees flexed and drop your feet from the left to the right as a counter movement to the backbend.

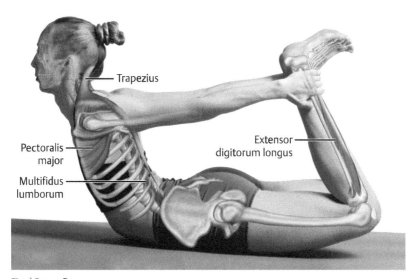

Trapezius

Pectoralis major

Multifidus lumborum

Extensor digitorum longus

Final Pose: **Bow**

Wheel
(Urdhva Dhanurasana)

Summary of the Pose

This challenging backbend stretches the chest, abdomen, and shoulders while strengthening the thighs and legs.

Modifications: Work on Bridge to build strength before trying the final expression of this pose. Try using a block between your thighs to prevent the lower limbs from abducting. Place a block under your sacrum in the prep poses for additional support if needed.

Guided Narrative

Transition 1: **Bridge**

- Begin supine. Triceps brachii extends your arms and forearms along the ground by the sides of your body, and then utilize pronator quadratus and pronator teres (**Fig. 10.12**) to pronate your forearms, pressing your palms into the mat.
- Use your hamstrings (**Fig. 11.4**) to flex at your knees bringing your feet to the ground close to your gluteal muscles. Ensure that your feet are hip-width distance apart and that your knee joints are directly superior to your ankle joints.
- Press into your feet to lift your hips, rolling up from your sacrum through your upper thoracic vertebrae. Contract trapezius and your rhomboids (**Fig. 10.2**) to retract your scapulae, and externally rotate your arms with the aid of infraspinatus and teres minor. Interlace your fingers if comfortable.
- Relax your gluteal muscles and work on engaging your hamstrings to extend and lift your hips. Use your abdominals (**Fig. 9.5**) to stabilize through your core.
- On an exhalation, release down to your back, one vertebra at a time from your cervical spine through your coccyx. Gently drop both knees to the right and to the left to counter release from this pose.

● ●

Transition 2: **Wheel Prep**

- Flex your arms up and over your head, and then flex your forearms using brachialis (**Fig. 10.10**) to bring your palms to the ground lateral to your ears with your fingers pointing toward your shoulders. Abduct your fingers using your dorsal interossei (**Fig. 10.15**).
- Press into your feet and roll from your sacrum to your thoracic vertebrae. With your hips lifted, press into your hands and feet to place the top of your skull on the mat.
- Contract pectoralis major to adduct your arms pointing your elbows straight up and adductor magnus (**Fig. 11.3**) to internally rotate your thighs.
- Ensure that your thighs are still parallel by activating gracilis and your adductors, visualizing the course of the obturator nerve passing through the obturator foramen to innervate these muscles.

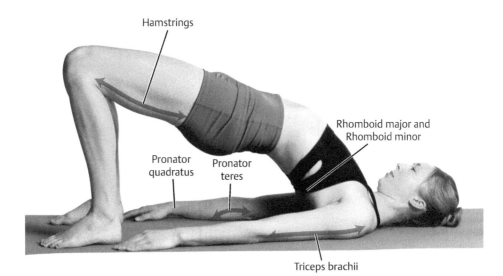

Hamstrings

Rhomboid major and
Rhomboid minor

Pronator
quadratus

Pronator
teres

Triceps brachii

Transition 1: **Bridge**

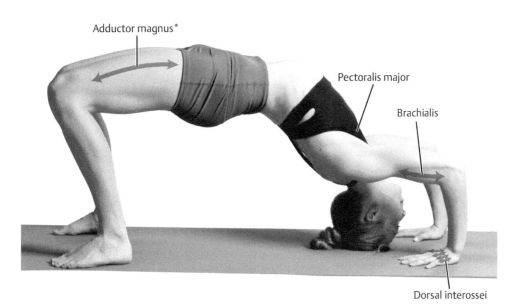

Adductor magnus*

Pectoralis major

Brachialis

Dorsal interossei

Transition 2: **Wheel Prep**

Final Pose: **Wheel**

- On an inhalation, press into your hands while extending your forearms using your triceps brachii (**Fig. 10.11**) and lift your pelvis to the ceiling.
- Keep your feet parallel and gradually work toward positioning your shoulder joints over your elbow joints. Feel deltoid working here to extend your shoulders and gluteus maximus to extend your hips.
- Continue to contract your erector spinae to extend through all regions of your vertebral column.
- Appreciate that teres minor and infraspinatus externally rotate your arms (**Fig. 10.4**), while gluteus medius and gluteus minimus (**Fig. 11.9**) internally rotate your thighs.
- Feel a stretch across deltoid (**Fig. 10.3**) and your abdominals, including your obliques.
- Exhale and flex your forearms and legs to lower down. First, place the back of your head on the ground and then roll down through each vertebra from the cervical region to the coccyx. Bring the soles of your feet to touch and your knees laterally to counter this pose (Reclined Bound Angle).

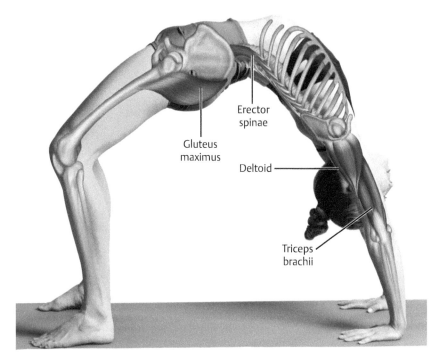

Erector spinae

Gluteus maximus

Deltoid

Triceps brachii

Final Pose: **Wheel**

5 Arm Balances

Downward Facing Dog
(Adho Mukha Svanasana)

Summary of the Pose

This is an important transition and resting pose in a yoga practice. It helps to stretch the posterior thighs and legs while also strengthening the arms and pectoral girdle. It is an excellent prep pose for other inversions.

Modifications: If you experience any wrist pain, place blocks underneath both hands. While in the second transition of this sequence, drop down to your knees, stack the shoulders over the wrists, and contract your abdominals until you cultivate the core strength required to hold the full expression.

Guided Narrative

Transition 1: **Table Top**

- Begin in Table Top by stacking your shoulders over your wrists and your hips over your knees.
- Use your triceps brachii (**Fig. 10.11**) to extend both elbows and your dorsal interossei of the hands (**Fig. 10.15**) to abduct and spread your fingers wide to create a strong base.
- From the innervation of your thoracoabdominal nerves (T7–T12) contract the muscles of your abdomen to stabilize your core.
- Notice that your hamstrings (**Fig. 11.13**) are working to flex both knees.
- Look a few inches in front of you to lengthen through your neck by contracting trapezius (**Fig. 10.2**).

•••

Transition 2: **Plank**

- Use your hamstrings to extend both your hips and quadriceps femoris (**Fig. 11.12**) to extend both knees pressing your toes into the mat behind you. Align your heels over your toes and your shoulders over your wrists.
- Press your heels to the back of the room and dorsiflex through your ankles recruiting the muscles of the anterior compartment of your legs, including tibialis anterior, extensor digitorum longus, and extensor hallucis longus (**Fig. 11.14**).
- Strongly press through your palms to protract your scapulae using serratus anterior (**Fig. 10.6**). Contract splenius capitis (**Fig. 8.2**) to look slightly forward maintaining the length in your neck.
- Muscles of the rotator cuff (**Fig. 10.4**) are helping to stabilize your shoulder joints here.
- Begin to strengthen your core finding a posterior pelvic tilt by drawing your pubic bone toward the top of your mat, engaging your rectus abdominis and transversus abdominis (**Fig. 9.7**).

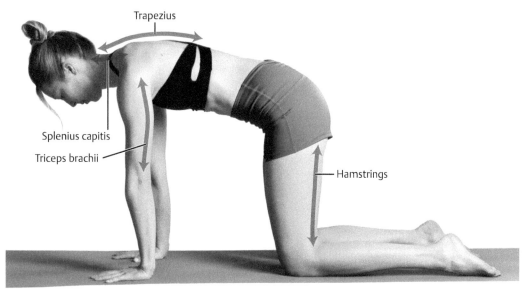

Trapezius

Splenius capitis

Triceps brachii

Hamstrings

Transition 1: **Table Top**

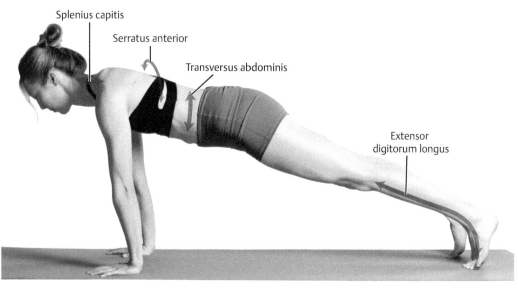

Splenius capitis

Serratus anterior

Transversus abdominis

Extensor digitorum longus

Transition 2: **Plank**

Final Pose: **Downward Facing Dog**

- While maintaining the placement of both hands, press into your palms to lift your hips. Work toward bringing your chest closer to the anterior surface of your thighs. Microbend your knees and direct your ischial tuberosities upward.
- Use your deltoid (**Fig. 10.3**) and the long head of biceps brachii (**Fig. 10.10**) to flex at the shoulder. Engage your triceps brachii to extend both elbows.
- Press firmly into both palms, specifically the lateral side of each hand, formed by the pollex and first digit. Notice that both of your forearms are pronated and your arms are laterally rotated.
- Turn both sets of toes in slightly to promote additional internal rotation of both femurs. Your adductor magnus (**Fig. 11.2**) will also help with this internal rotation and adduction.
- Feel your hamstrings and gastrocnemius muscles (**Fig. 11.16**) stretching in this pose. Option to flex deeply through one knee and then the other to stretch out the muscles of your calf before settling into the pose.
- Release the pose on an exhalation by flexing your knees, returning your patellae back to the mat in Table Top.

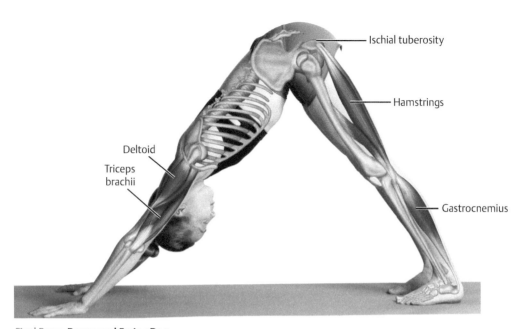

Ischial tuberosity

Hamstrings

Deltoid

Triceps
brachii

Gastrocnemius

Final Pose: **Downward Facing Dog**

Four-Limbed Staff
(Chaturanga Dandasana)

Summary of the Pose

Commonly found in many *vinyasa* yoga sequences, this pose strengthens the arms, core, thighs, and legs.

Modifications: Keep your knees on the ground in Plank and Four-Limbed Staff to gradually build strength working toward the full expression of the pose.

Guided Narrative

Transition 1: **Table Top**

- From a seated position, plant your palms onto the mat and extend your legs behind you, stacking your shoulders above your wrists and your hips above your knees.
- Use your triceps brachii (**Fig. 10.11**) to extend both elbows and your dorsal interossei of the hands (**Fig. 10.15**) to abduct and spread your fingers wide creating a firm base.
- Notice that your hamstrings (**Fig. 11.13**) are working to flex both knees.
- Lengthen from your coccyx through the crown of your head and cultivate stability through your core by contracting your abdominals.
- Look about six inches in front of you by contracting trapezius (**Fig. 10.2**), supplied by the spinal accessory nerve (CN XI), to create a neutral vertebral column.

• •

Transition 2: **Plank**

- Use your hamstrings to extend both hips and quadriceps femoris (**Fig. 11.12**) to extend both knees pressing your toes into the mat behind you. Align your heels over your toes and your shoulders over your wrists.
- Direct your heels to the back of the room and dorsiflex through your ankles using the muscles of the anterior compartment of your legs, including tibialis anterior, extensor digitorum longus, and extensor hallucis longus (**Fig. 11. 14**).
- Strongly press through your palms to protract your scapulae using serratus anterior (**Fig. 10.6**). Contract splenius capitis (**Fig. 8.2**) to look slightly forward, maintaining the length in your neck.
- Muscles of the rotator cuff (**Fig. 10.4**) are helping to stabilize your shoulder joints here.
- Begin to strengthen your core finding a posterior pelvic tilt by drawing your pubis toward the top of your mat, engaging your rectus abdominis and transversus abdominis muscles (**Fig. 9.7**).

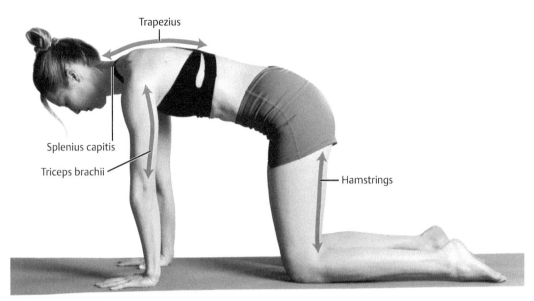

Trapezius

Splenius capitis

Triceps brachii

Hamstrings

Transition 1: **Table Top**

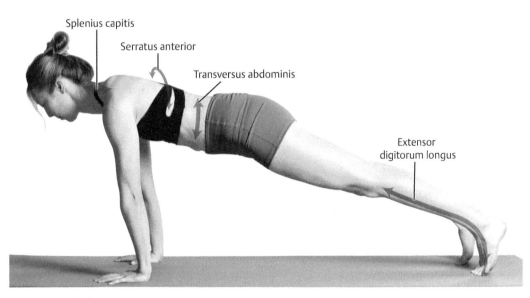

Splenius capitis

Serratus anterior

Transversus abdominis

Extensor digitorum longus

Transition 2: **Plank**

Final Pose: **Four-Limbed Staff**

- Inhale and hinge forward to stack your shoulders over your wrists. Exhale and use biceps brachii and brachialis (**Fig. 10.10**) to lower halfway, keeping your elbows close to your ribcage and flexed to no more than a 90-degree angle. Keep your gaze forward a few inches in front of your mat.
- Continue to engage rectus abdominis to further strengthen your core, your hamstrings to extend both hips, and your quadriceps femoris to extend both knees.
- Hug your elbows in medially continuing to retract your scapulae using rhomboid major and rhomboid minor.
- Stay active through the thighs, observing adductor magnus adducting and internally rotating your hips.
- If you feel unstable here, lower down to your patellae.
- Exit this pose on an exhalation by either: (1) shifting forward and rolling over the toes into Upward Facing Dog (see chapter 4), or (2) flexing your knees and sitting back on your heels in Child's Pose.

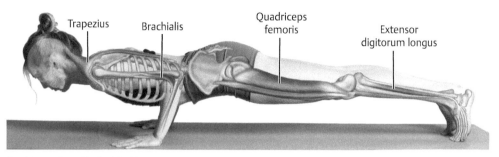

Trapezius

Brachialis

Quadriceps femoris

Extensor digitorum longus

Final Pose: **Four-Limbed Staff**

Side Plank
(Vasisthasana)

Summary of the Pose

Adding to the benefits of Plank, this variation strengthens your abdominal obliques and challenges your balance and alignment.

Modifications: Stay in Supported Side Plank (transition 2) until you gain enough strength for the final pose. Practice against a wall if you need support while balancing in this pose.

Guided Narrative

Transition 1: **Plank**

- From Table Top (see chapter 4, Camel, transition 1), use your hamstrings (**Fig. 11.13**) to extend both hips and quadriceps femoris (**Fig. 11.12**) to extend both knees pressing your toes into the mat behind you. Align your heels over your toes and your shoulders over your wrists.
- Press your heels to the back of the room and dorsiflex through your ankles utilizing the muscles of the anterior compartment of your leg, including tibialis anterior, extensor digitorum longus, and extensor hallucis longus (**Fig. 11.14**).
- Strongly press through your palms to protract your scapulae with the help of serratus anterior (**Fig. 10.6**). Contract splenius (**Fig. 8.2**) to look slightly forward maintaining the length of your neck.
- Muscles of the rotator cuff (**Fig. 10.4**) are helping to stabilize your shoulder joints here.
- Begin to strengthen your core finding a posterior pelvic tilt by drawing your pubis toward the top of your mat, engaging your rectus abdominis and transversus abdominis muscles (**Fig. 9.7**).

• •

Transition 2: **Supported Side Plank**

- Transfer weight onto your right hand while turning your torso to the left, activating your external and internal obliques and rectus abdominis (**Fig. 9.5**).
- Abduct your right thigh bringing your knee to the ground, using gluteus medius, gluteus minimus, and tensor fasciae latae (**Fig. 11.1** and **Fig. 11.6**), all of which receive branches from the superior gluteal nerve.
- Strongly push into the ground with your right palm, engaging triceps brachii to extend your forearm and serratus anterior to protract your scapula. Inhale and abduct your left arm out to the side and then over your head using deltoid (**Fig. 10.3**).
- Stack your left hip superior to your right and point your anterior superior iliac spines to the long edge of your mat.
- Gaze toward your left hand if comfortable in your neck or to the side of your mat.
- Lower your left palm down and return to plank. Repeat this pose on your left side.

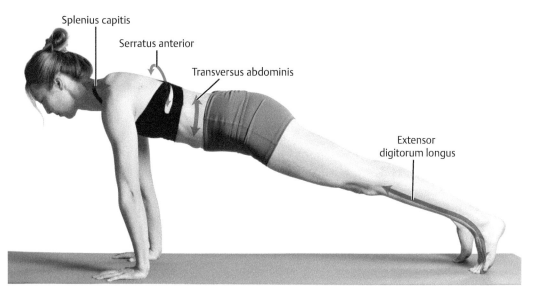

Splenius capitis

Serratus anterior

Transversus abdominis

Extensor digitorum longus

Transition 1: **Plank**

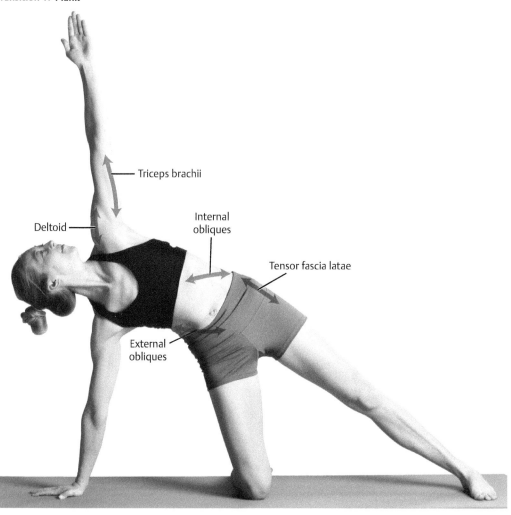

Triceps brachii

Deltoid

Internal obliques

Tensor fascia latae

External obliques

Transition 2: **Supported Side Plank.** Note: Tensor fascia latae is indicated on the opposite side than the text description for better visualization.

Final Pose: **Side Plank**

- From Supported Side Plank on your right hand, continue to engage your abdominals while you adduct your right thigh toward your left thigh and then use quadriceps femoris to extend your right leg to meet your left.
- Stack your left foot on top of your right foot, balancing on the lateral side of your fifth metatarsal and calcaneus. Continue to dorsiflex both feet using tibialis anterior. Option to bring your left foot anterior to your right foot for additional ankle stability.
- Create a long line from your calcanei through your lower limbs and up through your core. Align your right shoulder superior to your right wrist and rotate your left shoulder back to stack over your right shoulder.
- Avoid laterally flexing your vertebral column by lifting your hips too high.
- Option to lift your gaze toward your left hand through the unilateral action of your right sternocleidomastoid and your left splenius.
- Rotate your torso and lower your left hand down to plank. Repeat this pose on your left side.

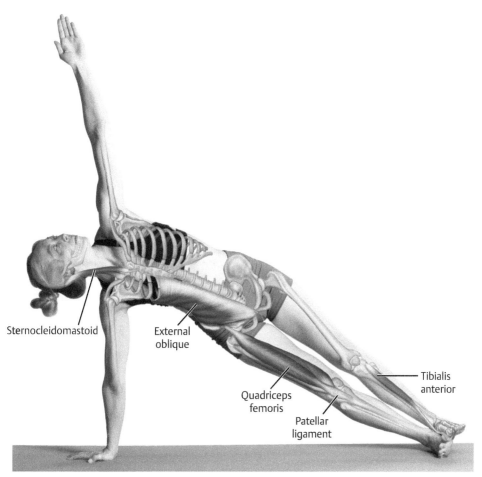

Sternocleidomastoid

External
oblique

Quadriceps
femoris

Patellar
ligament

Tibialis
anterior

Final Pose: **Side Plank**

Crow
(Kakasana)

Summary of the Pose

This is a foundational arm balancing posture that strengthens the shoulders, arms, forearms, hips, and core. It stretches the back and activates proprioceptors of the wrist to maintain balance. Note that when the forearms are extended, this pose is referred to as Crane (*Bakasana*).

Notes and Modifications: Place your feet on blocks or books and have a pillow on the ground in front of you for support. Place the feet on a wall behind you for additional stability as you gradually build the strength needed to support you in this pose.

Guided Narrative

Transition 1: **Garland**

- Begin standing with your feet wider than your hips and your toes pointing out.
- Sink into a low-squatting position by flexing your thighs while the hamstrings (**Fig. 11.13**) and gracilis (**Fig. 11.3**) flex your legs.
- Bring your palms together anterior to your sternum, hyperextending your wrists, using the muscles in the posterior compartment of the forearm (**Fig. 10.13**).
- Press your elbows into your thighs to encourage abduction of your hips.
- Slightly extend your spine, creating a straight line from the external occipital protuberance to the coccyx.

● ●

Transition 2: **Crow Prep**

- Pronate your forearms using pronator teres and pronator quadratus (**Fig. 10.12**), and extend your forearms activating triceps brachii (**Fig. 10.11**) to place your palms shoulder-distance apart on the mat in front of you. Abduct your fingers using your dorsal interossei (**Fig. 10.15**) to create as much surface area as possible to balance.
- Come to the balls of your feet by plantarflexing your ankles with the assistance of the muscles in the posterior compartment of your leg (**Fig. 11.16**).
- Create a shelf with your arms and forearms by contracting brachialis and pronator teres to flex your forearms at the elbows. Place your patellae on the lateral heads of triceps brachii and gaze slightly forward with trapezius.
- Begin flexing one leg off of the ground by contracting gastrocnemius and then plantarflex the foot at the ankle. Use quadriceps femoris (**Fig. 11.1**) to extend your leg, placing the foot back to the ground, and repeat this single leg lift on the other side.

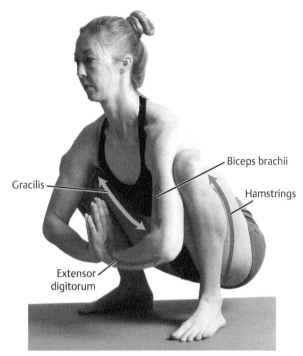

Gracilis

Biceps brachii

Hamstrings

Extensor
digitorum

Transition 1:   **Garland**

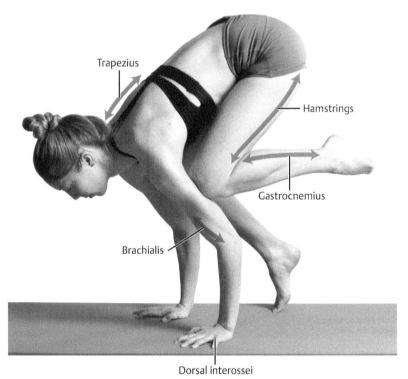

Trapezius

Hamstrings

Gastrocnemius

Brachialis

Dorsal interossei

Transition 2:   **Crow Prep**

Final Pose: **Crow**

- For the full expression of this pose, bilaterally flex both legs, one at a time, and plantarflex through the feet. Work toward placing your patellae close to your axilla.
- Grip the mat and push into the ground as you shift your weight forward. Feel serratus anterior (**Fig. 10.6**) protracting your scapulae and the abdominals strongly flexing your vertebral column, pulling your umbilicus up and into the core.
- Bilaterally contract trapezius, splenius capitis, and splenius cervicis (**Fig. 8.2**) to slightly extend the head, gazing a few inches in front of you.
- To release the pose, exhale and lower back to Garland (transition 1), then extend your legs, lift your hips, and exhale into a forward fold.

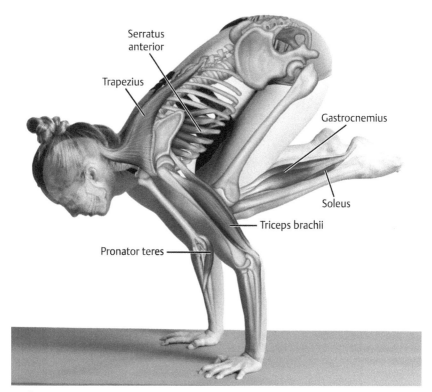

Serratus anterior

Trapezius

Gastrocnemius

Soleus

Triceps brachii

Pronator teres

Final Pose: **Crow**

6 Spinal Twists

Revolved Crescent Lunge
(Parivrtta Anjaneyasana)

Summary of the Pose

This is a variation of Crescent Lunge, which is often used as a transitional pose in *vinyasa* practices. This pose strengthens your legs and improves balance. The abdominal twist to the left compresses the ascending colon and twisting to the right compresses the descending colon.

Modifications: In all versions of this twist, you may flex your back knee down to the mat and place a blanket under the patella. In the final pose, you may place your hand on a block or book if it does not reach the mat. If pregnant, practice open twisting poses rather than deep twists.

Guided Narrative

Transition 1: Crescent Lunge

- From anatomical position, take a wide step back with your right foot into a high lunge position. Place the plantar surface of your right toes to the ground and work toward aligning your calcaneus over your metatarsals.
- Use your hamstrings (**Fig. 11.4**) in your front left leg to flex at the knee. Ensure that your knee joint stacks directly over your left ankle.
- Your gracilis, adductor longus, and adductor brevis (**Fig. 11.10**) are adducting your left thigh.
- Quadriceps femoris (**Fig. 11.1**) is engaged to extend your right leg to the back of your mat, while the hamstrings and gluteus maximus are working to extend your right thigh.
- Abduct your arms out to the sides and over your head by contracting supraspinatus and deltoid (**Fig. 10.2**), then extend your forearms parallel to each other using triceps brachii (**Fig. 10.11**).
- On your inhalations, reach upward and feel erector spinae (**Fig. 8.2**) extend your vertebral column. Sink deeper into your lunge on your exhalations.

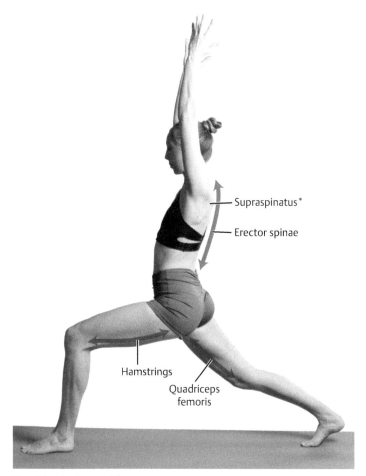

Supraspinatus*

Erector spinae

Hamstrings

Quadriceps
femoris

Transition 1: **Crescent Lunge**

Transition 2: **Revolved Crescent Prep**

- Use pectoralis major (**Fig. 10.5**) and latissimus dorsi (**Fig. 10.9**) to adduct your arms, pressing your palms together, then bring them down and anterior to your sternum.
- Feel your scapulae retract using rhomboid major, rhomboid minor, and the middle fibers of trapezius.
- Bring weight into your front left foot and begin to flex your torso forward using rectus abdominis (**Fig. 9.5**), keeping your hands at your sternum.
- Use your abdominals to rotate your torso bringing the lateral edge of your right elbow to the outside of your left thigh.
- Your left internal oblique and right external oblique are working to rotate your trunk to the side of your mat. This trunk rotation is also aided by the transversospinalis muscles (**Fig. 8.2**).
- With every inhalation, lengthen from the crown of your head to your sacrum and with every exhalation twist deeper.

• •

Final Pose: **Revolved Crescent**

- While inhaling, contract your left supraspinatus and deltoid to abduct your left arm up to the ceiling. Use your right triceps brachii to extend your right arm and then extend your forearm and wrist to place your hand down to the ground or block on the outside of your left foot. Press your right forearm into your left thigh or leg to deepen the twist.
- If comfortable, contract your right sternocleidomastoid and left splenius capitis and cervicis (**Fig. 8.2**) to turn your head to the left, gazing superiorly toward the ceiling.
- Using the muscles in both posterior compartments (**Fig. 10.11**), bilaterally extend both forearms and wrists in opposite directions.
- Continue to engage your hamstrings to flex and stabilize your front left knee to allow for a deeper lunge.
- Exhale as you twist deeper and feel the stretch in your external and internal intercostal muscles (**Fig. 9.4**) on your left side.
- On an exhalation, unwind from this twist by returning back to Crescent Lunge (transition 1), switch your stance, and repeat this sequence on the other side.

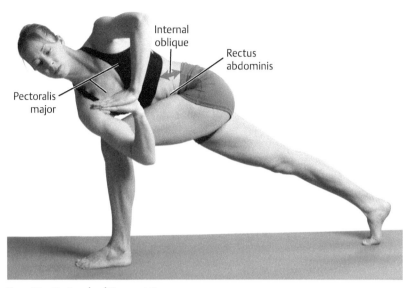

Transition 2: **Revolved Crescent Prep**

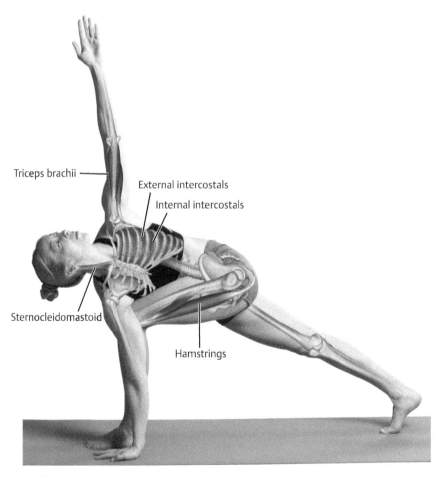

Final Pose: **Revolved Crescent**

Revolved Triangle
(Parivrtta Trikonasana)

Summary of the Pose

This pose adds a deep spinal twist to Triangle (see chapter 1, standing poses) and challenges the breath and balance. It stretches the hamstrings, calves, and ankles and stimulates the abdominal organs.

Modifications: Balancing in this pose may be challenging if your hamstrings are tight. Place your lower hand on a block or book if it does not reach the mat. Practice this pose against a wall for additional stability. If pregnant, practice open twisting poses rather than deep twists.

Guided Narrative

Transition 1: **Warrior I**

- Begin in Warrior I (see chapter 1, standing poses) by taking a large step back with the left foot and placing it at a 45-degree angle. Align your right calcaneus with your left calcaneus for heel-to-heel alignment.
- Contract your right hamstrings (**Fig. 11.4**) to flex your front leg and engage your left quadriceps femoris (**Fig. 11.1**) to extend your back leg. Use gracilis and adductor magnus (**Fig. 11.3**) to adduct both thighs toward the midline.
- Let suprapinatus and deltoid abduct your arms out to the sides and over your head. Extend both forearms with triceps brachii. Depress your scapulae using the ascending fibers of trapezius to draw your shoulders inferiorly down your back and away from your ears.
- On your inhalations, lift the upper body and contract your abdominals, feeling the support from rectus abdominis along the front of your core. Sink deeper into your lunge on your exhalations.

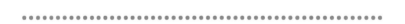

Transition 2: **Pyramid**

- Prepare for Pyramid (see chapter 3, forward folds) by stepping your left foot a few inches forward to shorten your stance, and then slightly internally rotate your back foot so that all of your toes point forward to the top of your mat.
- Bilaterally contract quadriceps femoris to extend your legs, straightening through both knee joints.
- Gently pull your right hip joint back and your left hip joint forward to align both of your anterior superior iliac spines to the front of your mat, squaring off your hips.
- Flex your vertebral column over your right thigh by contracting your abdominals (**Fig. 9.5**), iliacus, and psoas major (**Fig. 11.1**). Work toward drawing your chin toward your leg and place your hands to the ground or to blocks on either side of your front foot.
- Feel a stretch along the right hamstrings and muscles of the right posterior leg.

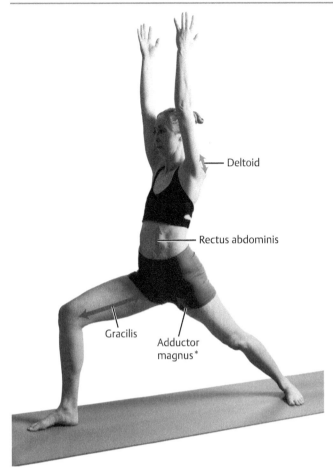

Deltoid

Rectus abdominis

Gracilis

Adductor magnus*

Transition 1: **Warrior I**

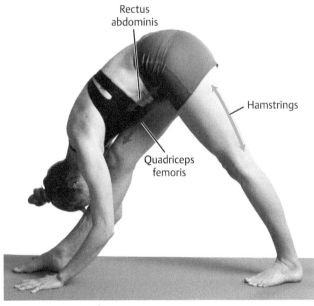

Rectus abdominis

Hamstrings

Quadriceps femoris

Transition 2: **Pyramid**

Final Pose: **Revolved Triangle**[1]

- Press your left hand into the floor outside of your front foot while contracting your left external oblique and right internal oblique to rotate your chest to the right. Abduct your right arm toward the ceiling.
- Contract triceps brachii to extend your right arm and utilize extensors of the forearm (**Fig. 10.13**) to extend your wrist and fingers.
- Feel the stretch across your chest as you retract your scapulae using the middle fibers of trapezius and your rhomboid major and rhomboid minor.
- Contract your left sternocleidomastoid and your right splenius muscles (**Fig. 10.2**) to turn your head to the right, gazing toward your lifted fingers.
- Inhale and lengthen from your skull to your coccyx. Exhale and continue to rotate your vertebral column to deepen the twist while keeping your hips squared to the front of the mat through the bilateral action of adductor magnus.
- Exhale while releasing your right hand back down to the mat and repeat this sequence on the other side.

---

[1]To better illustrate the twist, note that the model is in Revolved Triangle with her left foot forward while the description continues to instruct you with your right foot forward.

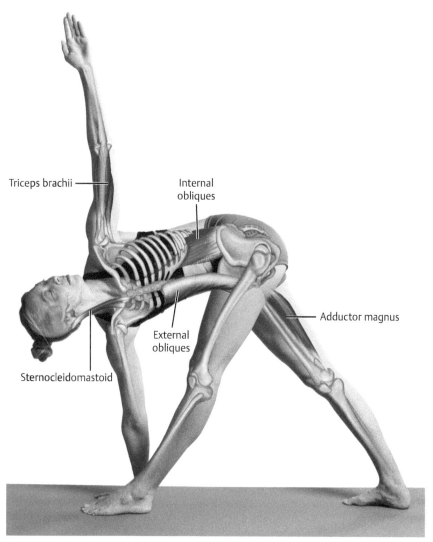

Triceps brachii

Internal obliques

Adductor magnus

External obliques

Sternocleidomastoid

Final Pose: **Revolved Triangle**

Half Lord of the Fishes
(Ardha Matsyendrasana)

Summary of the Pose

This seated twist helps to compress the abdominal organs, such as the liver and the kidneys. It stretches the shoulders, hips, and neck.

Modifications: Stay in any transition pose of this sequence until you gain the mobility to move deeper into the twist. If pregnant, practice open twisting poses rather than deep twists.

Guided Narrative

Transition 1: **Staff**

- From a seated position, use quadriceps femoris (**Fig. 11.1**) to extend both knees out in front of you.
- Press your hands into the mat on either side of your pelvis and extend both elbows with triceps brachii (**Fig. 10.11**).
- Contract tibialis anterior (**Fig. 11.14**) to dorsiflex both feet and use extensor digitorum longus and extensor hallucis longus to point your toes toward the ceiling.
- Feel grounded through both ischial tuberosities and engage your erector spinae (**Fig. 8.2**) to extend and lengthen your back.

• •

Transition 2: **Half Lord of the Fishes Prep 1**

- Begin to flex your left thigh to bring your knee to your chest, contracting your hip flexors including psoas major and iliacus (**Fig. 9.6**).
- Use you left hamstrings (**Fig. 11.4**) to flex your left leg to stamp your left foot firmly on the mat lateral to your right thigh. Remind yourself of the specific innervation of the hamstrings, with all components innervated by the tibial nerve, except for the short head of biceps femoris (which is innervated by the common fibular nerve).
- Continue to engage your right tibialis anterior to dorsiflex your right foot at the ankle, and extensor digitorum longus and extensor hallucis longus to extend through your right toes.
- Maintain the hyperextension of both wrists with the aid of extensor digitorum (**Fig. 10.13**) in the posterior compartment of the forearm.

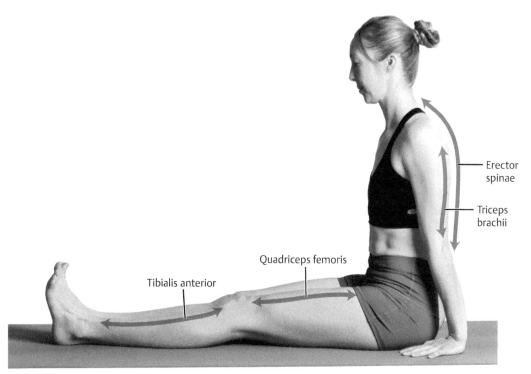

Transition 1: **Staff**

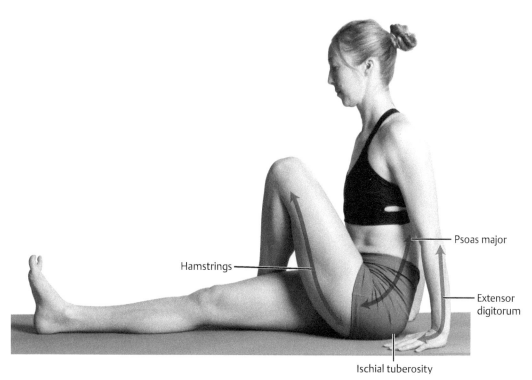

Transition 2: **Half Lord of the Fishes Prep 1**

Transition 3: **Half Lord of the Fishes Prep 2**

- Externally rotate your left arm utilizing infraspinatus and teres minor to bring your left palm behind you with your fingers pointing to the back of the mat. Observe that while both infraspinatus and teres minor produce the same action, they differ in innervation (suprascapular nerve and axillary nerve, respectively).
- Use your left triceps brachii to extend your forearm while your right biceps brachii flexes your elbow to hug your right knee close to your body.
- Contract your right sternocleidomastoid (**Fig. 9.1**) to rotate your head to the left and look towards the back of your mat if comfortable.
- Note that your left internal oblique muscles are helping you to twist to the left.
- On your inhalations, lengthen your vertebral column and ground down evenly through both ischial tuberosities. Twist deeper into this pose on your exhales as you pivot your chest and shoulders to the left side of the room.

Final Pose: **Half Lord of the Fishes**

- To enter a deeper variation of this twist, flex your right knee and use your hamstrings to bring your right foot close to your left gluteus maximus.
- Your right obturator internus and obturator externus are working to help you externally rotate your right hip. In addition, both sartorius muscles are helping to flex your hip and knee joints bilaterally.
- Use biceps brachii to flex your right arm and hook your right elbow to the lateral side of your left knee if possible. Supinate your right forearm as you twist; note that supinator is innervated by the deep radial nerve (**Fig. 10.13**).
- If comfortable for your neck, use your right sternocleidomastoid to rotate your head to the left side of your mat. As your gaze shifts back, feel a stretch across your left pectoralis major.
- Unwind from this twist on an exhalation, extend your legs long out in front of you, and repeat this sequence by flexing your right knee and twisting to the right.

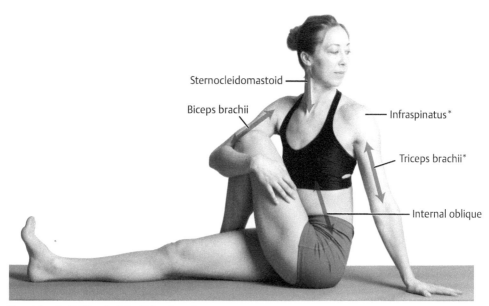

Sternocleidomastoid

Biceps brachii

Infraspinatus*

Triceps brachii*

Internal oblique

Transition 3: **Half Lord of the Fishes Prep 2**

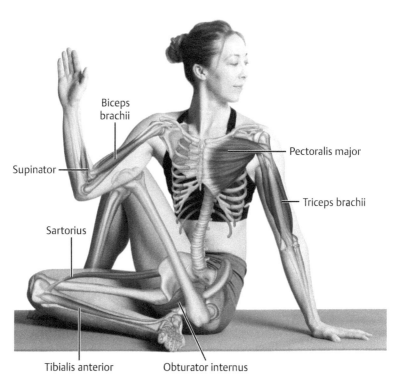

Biceps brachii

Pectoralis major

Supinator

Triceps brachii

Sartorius

Tibialis anterior

Obturator internus

Final Pose: **Half Lord of the Fishes**

Supine Twist
(Jathara Parivritti)

Summary of the Pose

This pose uses gravity to twist three regions of the vertebral column: cervical, thoracic, and lumbar. It also compresses three parts of the large intestine: ascending, transverse, and descending colons.

Modifications: Option to place a block or blanket between your thighs or under your knee during the twist for additional support. If pregnant, practice open twisting poses rather than deep twists.

Guided Narrative

Transition 1: **Wind Removing Pose**

- Begin supine and use both hamstrings (**Fig. 11.4**) to flex at the knees to draw them into your chest.
- Notice that you are using your right and left psoas major, iliacus, and rectus femoris (**Fig. 11.1**) to flex both hips.
- Use your biceps brachii (**Fig. 10.10**) to flex at both elbows to hug your forearms around your knees, compressing your upper abdomen and transverse colon.
- Continue to press your shoulders and back of your head into the mat.

• •

Transition 2: **Supine Twist Prep**

- Abduct both arms into a "T" shape and press your shoulders into the mat. Your palms can be either supinated or pronated.
- Use your abdominals to drop both knees over to the left with control, bringing your right hip to stack superior to your left hip. Your knees may touch, or a block or blanket can be placed between the knees.
- Feel your right gluteus maximus, right external and internal abdominal obliques stretch in this twist.
- Press your right shoulder down to further stretch your right pectoralis major. Use your left sternocleidomastoid to look over to the right if comfortable in the neck.
- After a few rounds of breath, strongly contract your abdominals to lift your knees up and over to the right side of the mat.

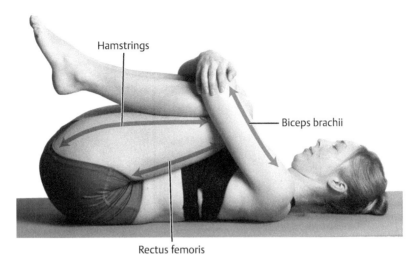

Hamstrings

Biceps brachii

Rectus femoris

Transition 1: **Wind Removing Pose**

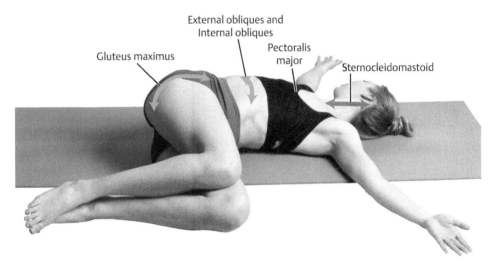

External obliques and
Internal obliques

Gluteus maximus

Pectoralis
major

Sternocleidomastoid

Transition 2: **Supine Twist Prep**

Final Pose: **Supine Twist**

- For this variation, from transition 2 with your knees to the left, extend your knees, being mindful of the femoral nerve innervating quadriceps femoris to extend both legs away from the mat.
- Use your left hand to draw your right knee closer to the ground, feeling the stretch in your right gluteus maximus, iliotibial band, and tensor fascia latae (**Fig. 11.6**) on your lateral right thigh.
- Use your left sternocleidomastoid and right splenius muscles to rotate your head to look over your right shoulder.
- Continue to press both shoulders into the mat, and use your exhalations to relax your body, allowing gravity to deepen the twist along your right side.
- Repeat this pose on the other side by first drawing your knees into your chest (transition 1) and then dropping your knees over to the right (transition 2) and extending your legs if you did this variation on the first side.

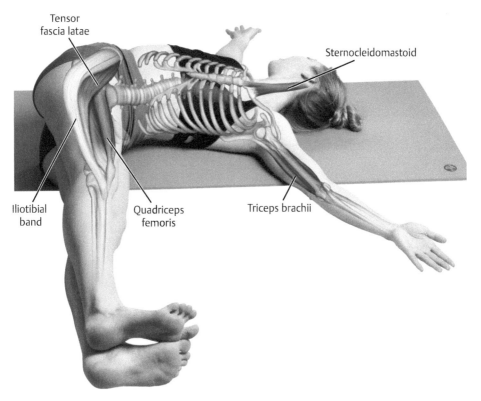

Tensor
fascia latae

Sternocleidomastoid

Iliotibial
band

Quadriceps
femoris

Triceps brachii

Final Pose: Supine Twist

7   Inversions

Bridge
(Setu Bandha Sarvangasana)

Summary of the Pose

Bridge provides a mild backbend to strengthen the hamstrings and back while stretching the muscles of the anterior thigh, pectoral region, and rotator cuff.

Modifications: Place a block under your sacrum for a supported variation of this pose.

Guided Narrative

Transition 1: **Bridge**

- Begin supine, using triceps brachii (**Fig. 10.11**) to extend your arms and forearms along the mat on either side of your abdomen. Contract pronator teres and pronator quadratus (**Fig. 10.12**) to place your palms on the ground.
- Flex your knees from the bilateral action of your hamstrings (**Fig. 11.13**) to place the plantar surface of your feet to the mat, approximately hips-width distance apart. Ensure that your knee joints are directly superior to your ankle joints.
- Press evenly into your feet and contract gluteus maximus (**Fig. 11.4**) and your hamstrings to extend your thighs, rolling up from your sacrum through your upper thoracic vertebrae.
- Maintain the same distance between your knee joints when lifting your hips using your adductors and gracilis (**Fig. 11.1**) to adduct your thighs.

Transition 2: **Bridge with Bind**

- Externally rotate both humeri by contracting teres minor, infraspinatus, and the posterior (spinal) part of deltoid (**Fig. 10.2**), and then retract your scapulae using rhomboids and the middle fibers of trapezius to roll your arms underneath you.
- Interlace your fingers and continue to extend your arms and forearms along the ground. Lift your sternum toward your mandible.
- To emphasize the work of your hamstrings, plantarflex both of your feet using gastrocnemius, soleus, and the deep flexors of the leg (**Fig. 11.16**) to rise onto your toes and lift your pubic bone toward the ceiling. While maintaining the lift of your hips, return your calcanei back down to the mat.

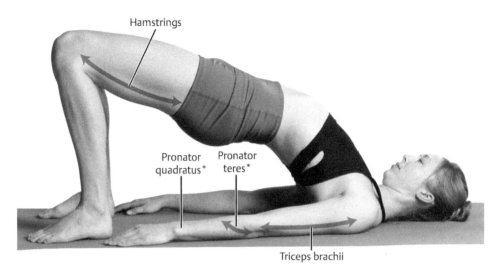

Hamstrings

Pronator
quadratus*

Pronator
teres*

Triceps brachii

Transition 1: **Bridge**

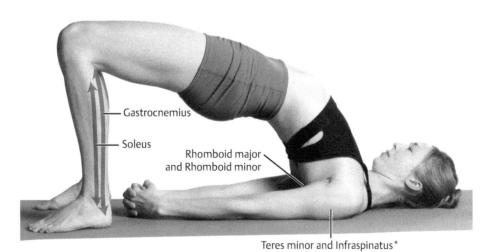

Gastrocnemius

Soleus

Rhomboid major
and Rhomboid minor

Teres minor and Infraspinatus*

Transition 2: **Bridge with Bind**

Final Pose: **Bridge with Extended Leg**

- If comfortable, enter a deeper variation of this pose by contracting psoas major and iliacus (**Fig. 9.6**) to flex your left thigh perpendicular to the mat. Then use quadriceps femoris (**Fig. 11.12**) to extend your left leg toward the ceiling.
- Practice bringing movement to the lifted ankle joint. First, dorsiflex your left foot by contracting the muscles of the anterior compartment of your leg (**Fig. 11.14**) so that the plantar surface of your foot is parallel to the ceiling. Then use the posterior compartment muscles (**Fig. 11.16**) to plantarflex the foot (as seen in the image).
- Continue to contract your right hamstrings to extend and lift the hips and press your forearms into the ground. These movements, along with contraction of erector spinae, deepen the extension of your back.
- Feel the stretch across your abdominals and pectoral muscles.
- On an exhalation, extend your left thigh and flex your leg to bring your left foot back down to the mat. Repeat this pose on the other side.
- To counter this pose, lie on your back and hug your knees into your chest, gently rocking from side to side to massage your low back.

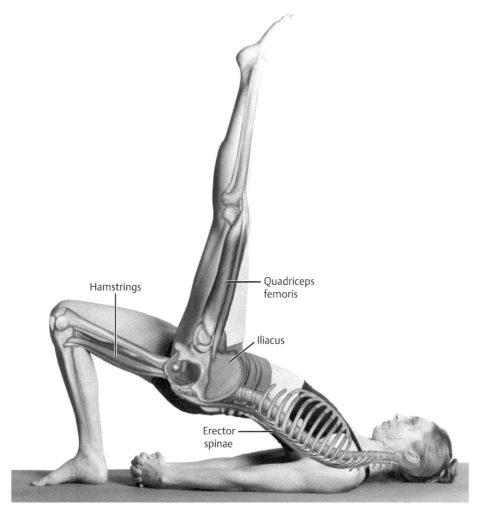

Final Pose: **Bridge with Extended Leg**

Hamstrings

Quadriceps
femoris

Iliacus

Erector
spinae

Supported Shoulder Stand and Plow
(Salamba Sarvangasana and Halasana)

Summary of the Pose

These supine inversions stretch the chest and shoulders and compress the neck viscera, including the thyroid gland (*jalandhara bandha*, throat lock). Some yoga philosophies believe shoulder stand helps calm the mind and regulates the cardiovascular and lymphatic systems.

Modifications: To help relieve pressure on the cervical spine in Shoulder Stand, try using two-folded blankets positioned lengthwise under your scapulae and rest your low back on a chair placed against a wall. If you are unable to bring your toes to the mat in Plow, place a block behind you.

Guided Narrative

Transition 1: **Shoulder Stand Prep**

- Begin lying supine with your legs extended along the ground. Place your palms to the mat next to your hips by pronating your forearms, contracting pronator teres and pronator quadratus (**Fig. 10.12**).
- Strongly contract your hip flexors to flex both thighs lifting your legs into the air. Use quadriceps femoris (**Fig. 11.12**) to extend your legs.
- Dorsiflex your feet at the ankles using the muscles of the anterior compartment of the leg.
- Draw your umbilicus in and upward to stabilize the core. Place a block under your sacrum for additional support to lift the hips in the next transition.

Transition 2: **Supported Shoulder Stand**

- Press into the ground and lift your hips upward and legs off of the mat. Use brachialis (**Fig. 10.10**) to flex your forearms and biceps brachii to flex and supinate your forearms bilaterally to bring your palms to your lumbar spine. One at a time, extend your thighs using your hamstrings (**Fig. 11.13**) and gluteus maximus (**Fig. 11.4**) to stack your hips inferior to your knee and ankle joints.
- Balance your weight on the tops of the shoulders, arms, elbows, and occiput.
- Plantarflex your ankles and then contract fibularis longus and fibularis brevis (**Fig. 11.15**) to slightly evert your foot at the ankle to point your toes straight upward. Note that these muscles of the lateral compartment of the leg are innervated by the superficial fibular nerve.
- Use your adductors, gracilis (**Fig. 11.3**), and pectineus (**Fig. 11.10**) to adduct the thighs toward the midline of your body.
- Contract rectus abdominis (**Fig. 9.5**) to vertically align the hip and shoulder joints. Avoid placing excessive pressure on the neck by maintaining the lordotic curvature, trying to keep the cervical vertebrae from touching the ground.

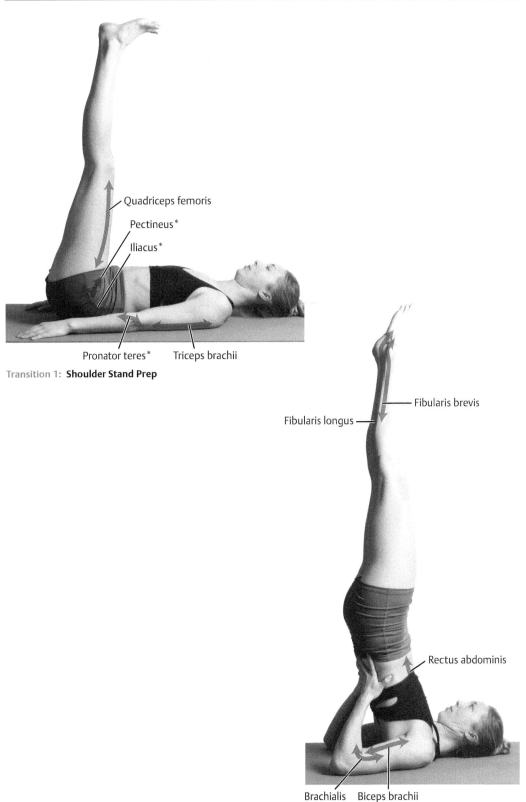

Quadriceps femoris

Pectineus*

Iliacus*

Pronator teres*   Triceps brachii

Transition 1: **Shoulder Stand Prep**

Fibularis brevis

Fibularis longus

Rectus abdominis

Brachialis   Biceps brachii

Transition 2: **Shoulder Stand**

115

Final Pose: **Plow**

- From Shoulder Stand, contract your hip flexors, including psoas major, to flex your thighs over your head while maintaining the extension of your legs. Strongly contract your abdominals, working toward bringing your toes to the back of your mat. If your hamstrings are tight and your feet do not reach the floor, place them on a block, a wall, or keep them hovering above the ground.
- Bilaterally extend both forearms using triceps brachii and anconeus (**Table 10.8**), both innervated by the radial nerve. Interlace your fingers, pressing the medial edge of your hands into the ground as seen in the image if comfortable.
- Continue to dorsiflex both feet at the ankles using extensor digitorum longus and fibularis tertius (**Fig. 11.14**) along with the other muscles of the anterior compartment.
- To exit this pose, bring your hands back to your sacrum, lift your legs to extend your thighs, and slowly roll back, one vertebra at a time, to a supine position.

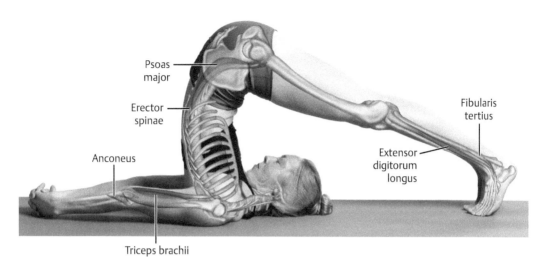

Psoas major

Erector spinae

Anconeus

Fibularis tertius

Extensor digitorum longus

Triceps brachii

Final Pose: **Plow**

Tripod Headstand
(Salamba Sirsasana II)

Summary of the Pose

This advanced inversion is a variation of traditional Headstand (*Salamba Sirsasana I*), in which the forearms are planted on the mat and fingers are interlaced behind the occipital bone. Headstand inversions strengthen the shoulders, tone the abdominal muscles, and are believed to aid the flow of blood and lymphatic fluid throughout the body.

Modifications: Fold your mat, place a blanket under your head, or place one block underneath each shoulder for additional support. Practice this pose against a wall or with a partner to spot you.

Guided Narrative

Transition 1: **Tripod Prep 1**

- Begin in Table Top (see chapter 4, Camel, transition 1) and ensure that your palms are shoulder-width distance apart. Abduct your fingers wide, contracting your dorsal interossei (Fig. 10.15), and hyperextend both wrists, activating your extensor digitorum (**Fig. 10.13**) in both forearms.
- Use both brachioradialis and brachialis (**Fig. 10.12**) to flex each elbow to a 90-degree angle.
- Engage your abdominal muscles, lift your hips, and begin to flex forward to bring the crown of your head to the mat, a few inches anterior to your fingertips.
- Plantarflex the ankles and begin to tiptoe your feet toward you activating quadriceps femoris (**Fig. 11.12**) to extend both knees working toward stacking your hip joints over your shoulder joints.
- Press weight evenly through both palms to avoid overengaging your neck muscles.
- Breathe while observing the stretch along your hamstrings and posterior leg compartment and the strength cultivated from your core and shoulders.

Transition 2: **Tripod Prep 2**

- From Tripod Prep 1, further engage psoas major and iliacus to flex your left hip and then use your hamstrings to flex your left knee placing it onto triceps brachii.
- With your left knee resting on your left triceps brachii, continue to ground down through your right toes to maintain balance.
- Begin to plantarflex your left foot by contracting your left soleus and gastrocnemius (**Fig. 11.16**).
- Continue to maintain stability in your shoulders by engaging teres major (**Fig. 10.11**) to adduct your arms.

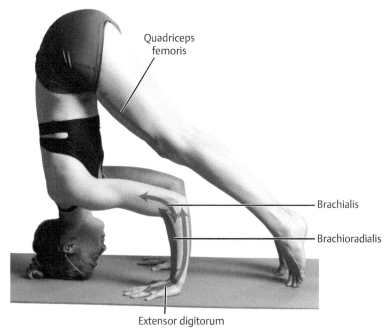

Quadriceps femoris

Brachialis

Brachioradialis

Extensor digitorum

Transition 1: **Tripod Prep 1**

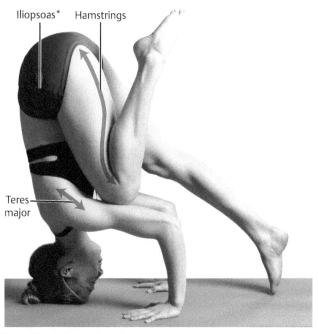

Iliopsoas*   Hamstrings

Teres major

Transition 2: **Tripod Prep 2**

Transition 3: **Tripod Prep 3**

- Only move onto this transition when you feel stable.
- Once stable, contract your right hamstrings and bring your right knee onto your right triceps brachii.
- Plantarflex both feet, utilizing the muscles of the posterior compartment of the legs.
- Engage your abdominal muscles (**Fig. 9.5**) and notice the bilateral contraction of latissimus dorsi to adduct your arms to maintain balance. Visualize the course of the thoracodorsal nerve emerging from the posterior cord of the brachial plexus as it innervates latissimus dorsi.
- While you will not feel them individually, the muscles of your suboccipital region (**Fig. 9.2**) are helping to stabilize your atlanto-axial and atlanto-occipital joints, which will help to prevent hypermobility of your neck.

Final Pose: **Tripod Headstand**

- Once you have gained strength and flexibility from the preparatory poses overtime, transition to Tripod Headstand.
- Press into both palms and contract gluteus maximus and your hamstrings (**Fig. 11.4**) to extend one thigh and then the other to stack your knees over your hip joints.
- Quadriceps femoris extends your legs to lift your feet upward. Plantarflex your ankles utilizing the posterior compartment of your leg.
- With both legs raised, engage your gracilis and adductor muscles (**Fig. 11.10**) to squeeze your thighs together. To maintain balance, engage rectus abdominis.
- To exit the pose, flex one hip at a time to bring your knees back to rest on your triceps brachii (transition 3). Bring both knees to the mat and push back into child's pose to rest and neutralize your spine.

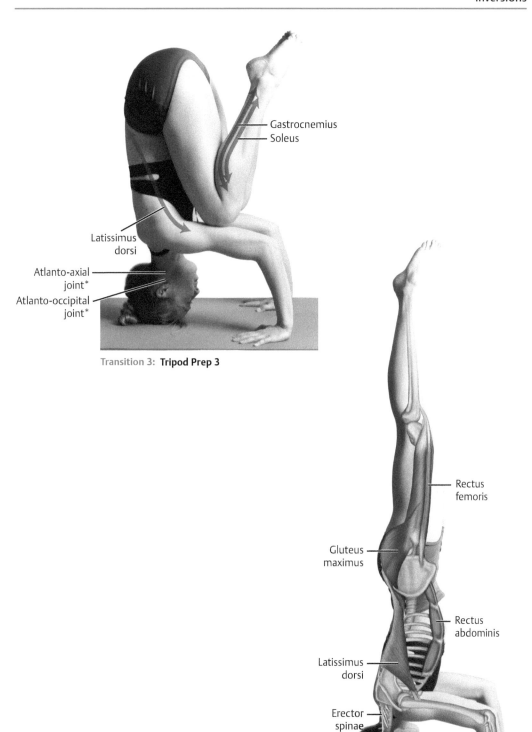

Gastrocnemius
Soleus
Latissimus dorsi
Atlanto-axial joint*
Atlanto-occipital joint*

Transition 3: **Tripod Prep 3**

Rectus femoris
Gluteus maximus
Rectus abdominis
Latissimus dorsi
Erector spinae

Final Pose: **Tripod Headstand**

Feathered Peacock (Forearm Stand)
(Pincha Mayurasana)

Summary of the Pose

This pose is a challenging arm balance which helps to strengthen the core and the upper body. Cultivate the strength and flexibility required for the final expression of this pose gradually over time with the preparatory postures in this sequence.

Modifications: Practice this pose against a wall for more support. Place a block between your palms to encourage the feeling of adduction in your arms to aid with stability.

Guided Narrative

Transition 1: **Downward Facing Dog**

- From a high push-up position, maintain the placement of both hands and feet and shift your weight backward. Press into your palms and lift your hips, working to bring your chest closer to the anterior surface of your thighs. Microbend your knees and direct your ischial tuberosities upward.
- While lifting your hips up and back, notice the use of your deltoid and biceps brachii (**Fig. 10.1**) to flex your shoulders, and triceps brachii (**Fig. 10.11**) to extend both elbows.
- Press firmly through both palms, specifically the lateral side of each hand, formed by the pollex and first digit. Observe the pronation of your forearm in this pose.
- Turn all of your toes in slightly to promote additional internal rotation of both femurs. Your adductor magnus (**Table 11.3**) will also help with this internal rotation and adduction.
- Feel your hamstrings and gastrocnemius (**Fig. 11.4**) stretching in this pose.

• •

Transition 2: **Dolphin**

- Flex your elbows, contracting brachialis and brachioradialis to lower onto your forearms. Press your palms into your mat or interlace your fingers into a fist.
- Hinge forward to bring your shoulders to stack superior to your elbows and begin walking your feet closer to your body. Utilize teres minor and infraspinatus (**Fig. 10.4**) to externally rotate both arms.
- Actively press your forearms into the mat and use pectoralis major to adduct your arms. Note that pectoralis major receives dual innervation from the medial and lateral pectoral nerves (**Table 10.3**).
- The muscles of your suboccipital triangle (**Fig. 9.2**) are important for proprioception as well as stabilizing and extending your neck to lift your head above the ground.
- As you walk your feet in closer, feel the stretch along the posterior compartments of your thighs and legs.

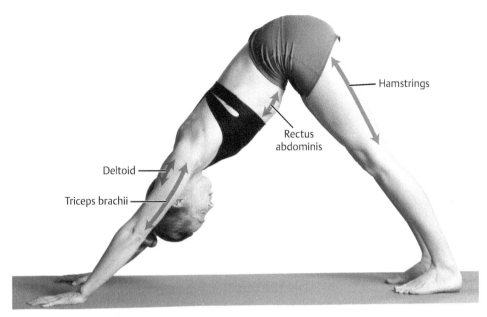

Hamstrings

Rectus abdominis

Deltoid

Triceps brachii

Transition 1: **Downward Facing Dog**

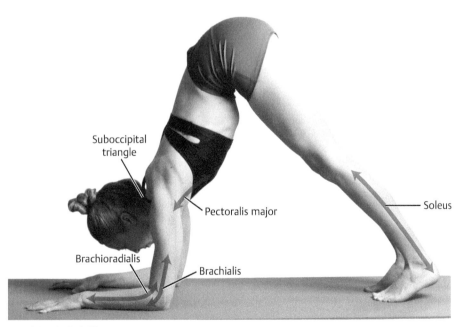

Suboccipital triangle

Pectoralis major

Soleus

Brachioradialis

Brachialis

Transition 2: **Dolphin**

Transition 3: **Feathered Peacock Prep**

- Prepare for Forearm Stand by contracting gluteus maximus and your hamstrings to extend your left foot upward with control. Once lifted, activate quadriceps femoris to extend your left leg and then plantarflex through your foot.
- Observe the opposing actions of extension in your left hip and flexion in your right hip from the contraction of your right psoas major and iliacus (**Fig. 9.6**).
- Promote stability in your shoulder girdles by pressing your palms and forearms firmly into your mat or the sides of a block, engaging pronator teres and pronator quadratus (**Fig. 10.12**).
- As you push into the ground, acknowledge serratus anterior (**Fig. 10.6**) working to protract and upwardly rotate both scapulae.
- On an exhalation, slowly flex your left thigh to bring your left foot to the mat. Repeat this prep pose on the other side, engaging your core to help maintain balance.

• •

Final Pose: **Feathered Peacock**

- For the full expression of this pose, strongly extend through your entire left leg to lift it upward and strongly contract your abdominals to take a small hop extending your right leg.
- Practice this light hop until you find balance on your forearms with both feet lifted off of the ground. Once you maintain balance, use quadriceps femoris (**Fig. 11.12**) to extend both knees toward the ceiling. Imagine stamping the plantar surface of your feet to the ceiling, feeling the dorsiflexion in your ankles.
- Engage your adductor muscles (**Fig. 11.10**) to help adduct your thighs together.
- Feel your abdominal muscles and psoas major contract to help stabilize the spine and prevent overextension of your lumbar vertebrae.
- To release, slowly flex one thigh and then the other returning to Dolphin (transition 2), and then drop down to your knees and rest in child's pose.

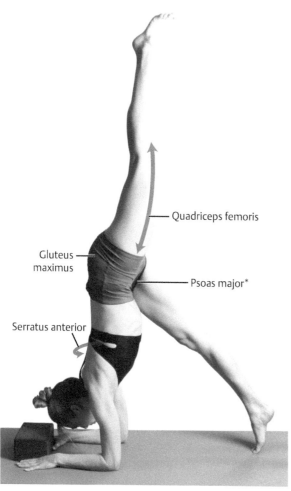

Quadriceps femoris

Gluteus maximus

Psoas major*

Serratus anterior

Transition 3: Feathered Peacock Prep

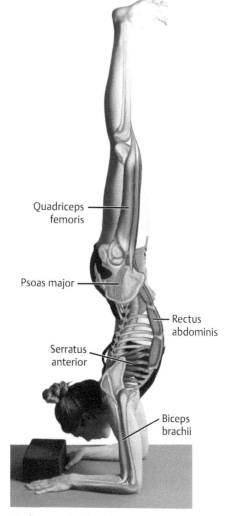

Quadriceps femoris

Psoas major

Rectus abdominis

Serratus anterior

Biceps brachii

Final Pose: Feathered Peacock

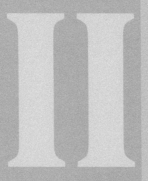

Part II
Yoga Anatomy

II

8 Back

Muscles of the Back

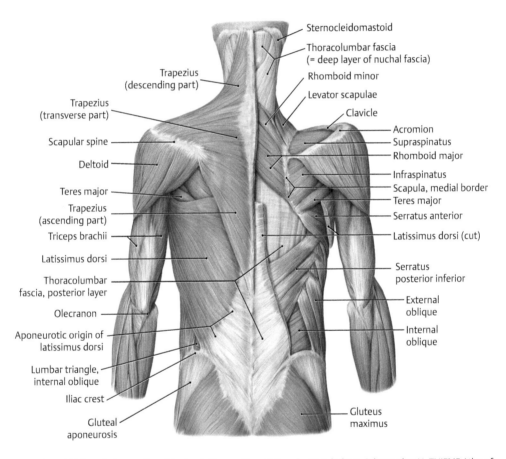

Fig. 8.1 Superficial extrinsic muscles of the back. Source: From Schuenke M, Schulte E, Schumacher U. THIEME Atlas of Anatomy. General Anatomy and Musculoskeletal System. Illustrations by Voll M and Wesker K. 2nd ed. New York: Thieme Medical Publishers; 2014.

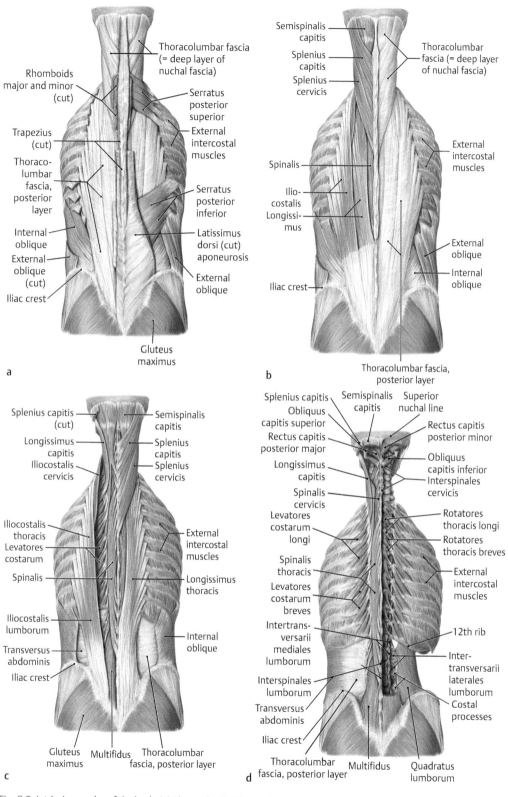

Fig. 8.2 Intrinsic muscles of the back. (a) Thoracolumbar fascia. (b) Superficial and intermediate intrinsic back muscles. (c) Intermediate and deep intrinsic back muscles. (d) Deep intrinsic back muscles. Source: From Schuenke M, Schulte E, Schumacher U. THIEME Atlas of Anatomy. General Anatomy and Musculoskeletal System. Illustrations by Voll M and Wesker K. 2nd ed. New York: Thieme Medical Publishers; 2014.

Table 8.1 Superficial intrinsic back muscles

Muscle		Origin	Insertion	Innervation	Action
Serratus posterior	Serratus posterior superior	Nuchal lig.; C7–T3 (spinous processes)	2nd–4th ribs (superior borders)	Spinal nn. T2–T5 (anterior rami)	Elevates ribs
	Serratus posterior inferior	T11–L2 (spinous processes)	8th–12th ribs (inferior borders, near angles)	Spinal nn. T9–T12 (anterior rami)	Depresses ribs
Splenius	Splenius capitis	Nuchal lig.; C7–T3 or T4 (spinous processes)	Lateral 1/3 nuchal line (occipital bone); mastoid process (temporal bone)	Spinal nn. C1–C6 (posterior rami, lateral branches)	*Bilateral:* Extends cervical spine and head *Unilateral:* Flexes and rotates head to the same side
	Splenius cervicis	T3–T6 or T7 (spinous processes)	C1–C3/4 (transverse processes)		

Source: From Gilroy AM et al. Atlas of Anatomy. 3rd ed. 2016. Based on: Schuenke M, Schulte E, Schumacher U. THIEME Atlas of Anatomy. General Anatomy and Musculoskeletal System. Illustrations by Voll M and Wesker K. 2nd ed. New York: Thieme Medical Publishers; 2014.

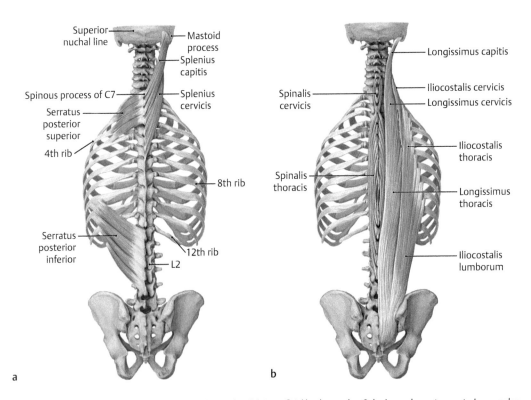

Fig. 8.3 Superficial and intermediate intrinsic back muscles. (**a**) Superficial back muscles: Splenius and serratus posterior muscles. (**b**) Intermediate intrinsic back muscles (erector spinae): Iliocostalis, longissimus, and spinalis muscles. Source: From Gilroy AM et al. Atlas of Anatomy. 3rd ed. 2016. Based on: Schuenke M, Schulte E, Schumacher U. THIEME Atlas of Anatomy. General Anatomy and Musculoskeletal System. Illustrations by Voll M and Wesker K. 2nd ed. New York: Thieme Medical Publishers; 2014.

Table 8.2 Intermediate intrinsic back muscles (erector spinae)

Muscle		Origin	Insertion	Innervation	Action
Iliocostalis	Iliocostalis cervicis	3rd–7th ribs	C4–C6 (transverse processes)	Spinal nn. C8–L1 (posterior rami, lateral branches)	*Bilateral:* Extends spine *Unilateral:* Bends spine laterally to same side
	Iliocostalis thoracis	7th–12th ribs	1st–6th ribs		
	Iliocostalis lumborum	Sacrum; iliac crest; thoracolumbar fascia (posterior layer)	6th–12th ribs; thoracolumbar fascia (posterior layer); upper lumbar vertebrae (transverse processes)		
Longissimus	Longissimus capitis	T1–T3 (transverse processes); C4–C7 (transverse and articular processes)	Temporal bone (mastoid process)	Spinal nn. C1–L5 (posterior rami, lateral branches)	*Bilateral:* Extends head *Unilateral:* Flexes and rotates head to same side
	Longissimus cervicis	T1–T6 (transverse processes)	C2–C5 (transverse processes)		
	Longissimus thoracis	Sacrum; iliac crest; lumbar vertebrae (spinous processes); lower thoracic vertebrae (transverse processes)	2nd–12th ribs; thoracic and lumbar vertebrae (transverse processes)		*Bilateral:* Extends spine *Unilateral:* Bends spine laterally to same side
Spinalis	Spinalis cervicis	C5–T2 (spinous processes)	C2–C5 (spinous processes)	Spinal nn. (posterior rami)	*Bilateral:* Extends cervical and thoracic spine *Unilateral:* Bends cervical and thoracic spine to same side
	Spinalis thoracis	T10–L3 (spinous processes, lateral surfaces)	T2–T8 (spinous processes, lateral surfaces)		

Source: From Gilroy AM et al. Atlas of Anatomy. 3rd ed. 2016. Based on: Schuenke M, Schulte E, Schumacher U. THIEME Atlas of Anatomy. General Anatomy and Musculoskeletal System. Illustrations by Voll M and Wesker K. 2nd ed. New York: Thieme Medical Publishers; 2014.

Table 8.3 Transversospinalis muscles

Muscle		Origin	Insertion	Innervation	Action
Rotatores	Rotatores breves	T1–T12 (between transverse and spinous processes of adjacent vertebrae)			*Bilateral:* Extends thoracic spine *Unilateral:* Rotates thoracic spine to opposite side
	Rotatores longi	T1–T12 (between transverse and spinous processes, skipping one vertebra)			*Bilateral:* Extends spine *Unilateral:* Flexes spine to same side, rotates it to opposite side
Multifidus		Sacrum, ilium, mamillary processes of L1–L5, transverse and articular processes of T1–T4, C4–C7	Superomedially to spinous processes, skipping two to four vertebrae	Spinal nn. (posterior rami)	
Semispinalis	Semispinalis capitis	C4–T7 (transverse and articular processes)	Occipital bone (between superior and inferior nuchal lines)		*Bilateral:* Extends thoracic and cervical spines and head (stabilizes craniovertebral joints)
	Semispinalis cervicis	T1–T6 (transverse processes)	C2–C5 (spinous processes)		*Unilateral:* Bends head, cervical and thoracic spines to same side, rotates to opposite side
	Semispinalis thoracis	T6–T12 (transverse processes)	C6–T4 (spinous processes)		

Source: From Gilroy AM et al. Atlas of Anatomy. 3rd ed. 2016. Based on: Schuenke M, Schulte E, Schumacher U. THIEME Atlas of Anatomy. General Anatomy and Musculoskeletal System. Illustrations by Voll M and Wesker K. 2nd ed. New York: Thieme Medical Publishers; 2014.

9 Neck, Thorax, and Abdomen

Muscles of the Neck

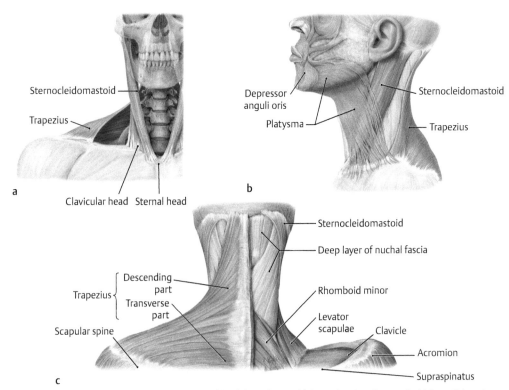

Fig. 9.1 Superficial neck muscles. (**a**) Anterior view. (**b**) Left lateral view. (**c**) Posterior view. Source: (a, b) From Schuenke M, Schulte E, Schumacher U. THIEME Atlas of Anatomy. General Anatomy and Musculoskeletal System. Illustrations by Voll M and Wesker K. 2nd ed. New York: Thieme Medical Publishers; 2014. (c) From Gilroy AM et al. Atlas of Anatomy. 3rd ed. 2016. Based on: Schuenke M, Schulte E, Schumacher U. THIEME Atlas of Anatomy. General Anatomy and Musculoskeletal System. Illustrations by Voll M and Wesker K. 2nd ed. New York: Thieme Medical Publishers; 2014.

Table 9.1 Superficial neck muscles

Muscle		Origin	Insertion	Innervation	Action
Platysma		Skin over lower neck and upper lateral thorax	Mandible (inferior border), skin over lower face and angle of mouth	Cervical branch of facial n. (CN VII)	Depresses and wrinkles skin of lower face and mouth, tenses skin of neck, aids forced depression of mandible
Sternoclei-domastoid	Sternal head	Sternum (manubrium)	Temporal bone (mastoid process), occipital bone (superior nuchal line)	*Motor:* Accessory n. (CN XI)	*Unilateral:* Tilts head to same side, rotates head to opposite side *Bilateral:* Extends head, aids in respiration when head is fixed
	Clavicular head	Clavicle (medial one third)		*Pain and proprioception:* Cervical plexus (C3, C4)	
Trapezius	Descending part	Occipital bone, spinous processes of C1–C7	Clavicle (lateral one third)		Draws scapula obliquely upward, rotates glenoid cavity superiorly

Source: From Gilroy AM et al. Atlas of Anatomy. 3rd ed. 2016. Based on: Schuenke M, Schulte E, Schumacher U. THIEME Atlas of Anatomy. General Anatomy and Musculoskeletal System. Illustrations by Voll M and Wesker K. 2nd ed. New York: Thieme Medical Publishers; 2014.

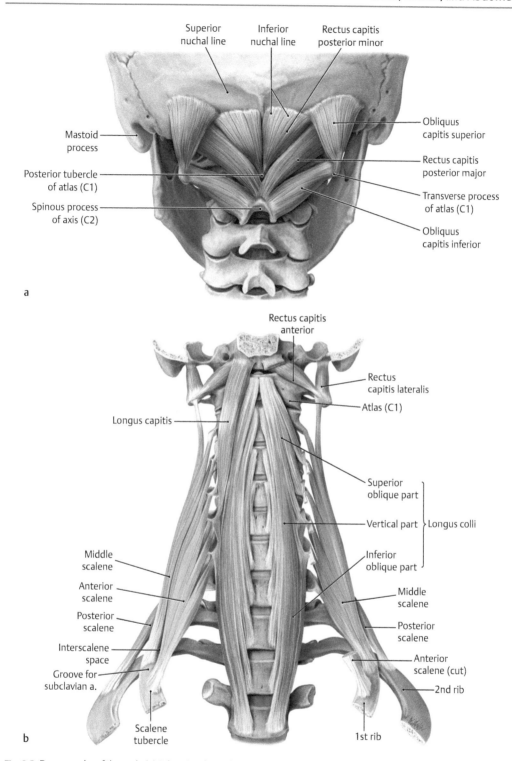

Fig. 9.2 Deep muscles of the neck. (**a**) Suboccipital muscles, posterior view. (**b**) Prevertebral and scalene muscles, anterior view. Source: From Schuenke M, Schulte E, Schumacher U. THIEME Atlas of Anatomy. General Anatomy and Musculoskeletal System. Illustrations by Voll M and Wesker K. 2nd ed. New York: Thieme Medical Publishers; 2014.

Table 9.2 Deep muscles of the neck

Muscle		Origin	Insertion	Innervation	Action
Prevertebral muscles					
Longus capitis		C3–C6 (anterior tubercles of transverse processes)	Occipital bone (basilar part)	Anterior rami of C1–C3	Flexion of head at atlanto-occipital joints
Longus colli	Vertical (intermediate) part	C5–T3 (anterior surfaces of vertebral bodies)	C2–C4 (anterior surfaces)	Anterior rami of C1–C6	*Unilateral:* Tilts and rotates cervical spine to opposite side

Bilateral: Forward flexion of cervical spine |
| | Superior oblique part | C3–C5 (anterior tubercles of transverse processes) | Atlas (anterior tubercle | | |
| | Inferior oblique part | T1–T3 (anterior surfaces of vertebral bodies) | C5–C6 (anterior tubercles of transverse processes) | | |
| Rectus capitis anterior | | C1 (lateral mass) | Occipital bone (basilar part) | Anterior rami of C1 and C2 | *Unilateral:* Lateral flexion of the head at the atlanto-occipital joint

Bilateral: Flexion of the head at the atlanto-occipital joint |
| Rectus capitis lateralis | | C1 (transverse process) | Occipital bone (basilar part, lateral to occipital condyles) | | |
| **Scalene muscles** | | | | | |
| Anterior scalene | | C3–C6 (anterior tubercles of transverse processes) | 1st rib (scalene tubercle) | Anterior rami of C4–C6 | *With ribs mobile:* Elevates upper ribs (during forced inspiration)

With ribs fixed: Bends cervical spine to same side (unilateral), flexes neck (bilateral) |
Middle scalene		C1–C2 (transverse processes), C3–C7 (posterior tubercles of transverse processes)	1st rib (posterior to groove for subclavian a.)	Anterior rami of C3–C8	
Posterior scalene		C5–C7 (posterior tubercles of transverse processes)	2nd rib (outer surface)	Anterior rami of C6–C8	
Suboccipital muscles (short nuchal and craniovertebral joint muscles)					
Rectus capitis posterior minor		C1 (posterior tubercle)	Occipital bone (inner third of inferior nuchal line)	Posterior ramus of C1 (suboccipital n.)	*Unilateral:* Rotates head to same side

Bilateral: Extends head |
| Rectus capitis posterior major | | C2 (spinous process) | Occipital bone (middle third of inferior nuchal line) | | |
| Obliquus capitis inferior | | | C1 (transverse process) | | |
| Obliquus capitis superior | | C1 (transverse process) | Occipital bone (above insertion of rectus capitis posterior major) | | *Unilateral:* Tilts head to same side, rotates it to opposite side

Bilateral: Extends head |

Source: From Gilroy AM et al. Atlas of Anatomy. 3rd ed. 2016. Based on: Schuenke M, Schulte E, Schumacher U. THIEME Atlas of Anatomy. General Anatomy and Musculoskeletal System. Illustrations by Voll M and Wesker K. 2nd ed. New York: Thieme Medical Publishers; 2014.

Muscles of the Thorax

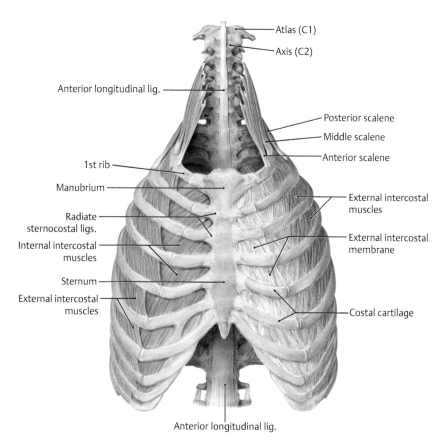

Fig. 9.3 Muscles of the thoracic wall, anterior view. Source: From Schuenke M, Schulte E, Schumacher U. THIEME Atlas of Anatomy. General Anatomy and Musculoskeletal System. Illustrations by Voll M and Wesker K. 2nd ed. New York: Thieme Medical Publishers; 2014.

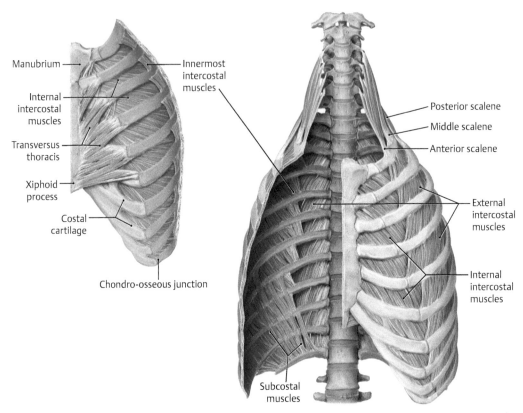

Fig. 9.4 Transversus thoracis. Source: From Gilroy AM et al. Atlas of Anatomy. 3rd ed. 2016. Based on: Schuenke M, Schulte E, Schumacher U. THIEME Atlas of Anatomy. General Anatomy and Musculoskeletal System. Illustrations by Voll M and Wesker K. 2nd ed. New York: Thieme Medical Publishers; 2014.

Table 9.3 Muscles of the thoracic wall

Muscle		Origin	Insertion	Innervation	Action
Scalene mm.	Anterior scalene m.	C3–C6 (transverse processes, anterior tubercles)	1st rib (anterior scalene tubercle)	Anterior rami of C4–C6 spinal nn.	*With ribs mobile:* Raises upper ribs (inspiration)
	Middle scalene m.	C3–C7 (transverse processes, posterior tubercles)	1st rib (posterior to groove for subclavian a.)	Anterior rami of C3–C8 spinal nn.	*With ribs fixed:* Bends cervical spine to same side (unilateral); flexes neck (bilateral)
	Posterior scalene m.	C5–C7 (transverse processes, posterior tubercles)	2nd rib (outer surface)	Anterior rami of C6–C8 spinal nn.	
Intercostal mm.	External intercostal mm.	Lower margin of rib to upper margin of next lower rib (courses obliquely forward and downward from costal tubercle to chondro-osseous junction)		1st to 11th intercostal nn.	Raises ribs (inspiration); supports intercostal spaces; stabilizes chest wall
	Internal intercostal mm.	Lower margin of rib to upper margin of next lower rib (courses obliquely forward and upward from costal angle to sternum)			Lowers ribs (expiration); supports intercostal spaces, stabilizes chest wall
	Innermost intercostal mm.				
Subcostal mm.		Lower margin of lower ribs to inner surface of ribs two to three ribs below		Adjacent intercostal nn.	Lowers ribs (expiration)
Transversus thoracis m.		Sternum and xiphoid process (inner surface)	2nd to 6th ribs (costal cartilage, inner surface)	2nd to 6th intercostal nn.	Weakly lowers ribs (expiration)

Source: From Gilroy AM et al. Atlas of Anatomy. 3rd ed. 2016. Based on: Schuenke M, Schulte E, Schumacher U. THIEME Atlas of Anatomy. General Anatomy and Musculoskeletal System. Illustrations by Voll M and Wesker K. 2nd ed. New York: Thieme Medical Publishers; 2014.

Muscles of the Abdomen

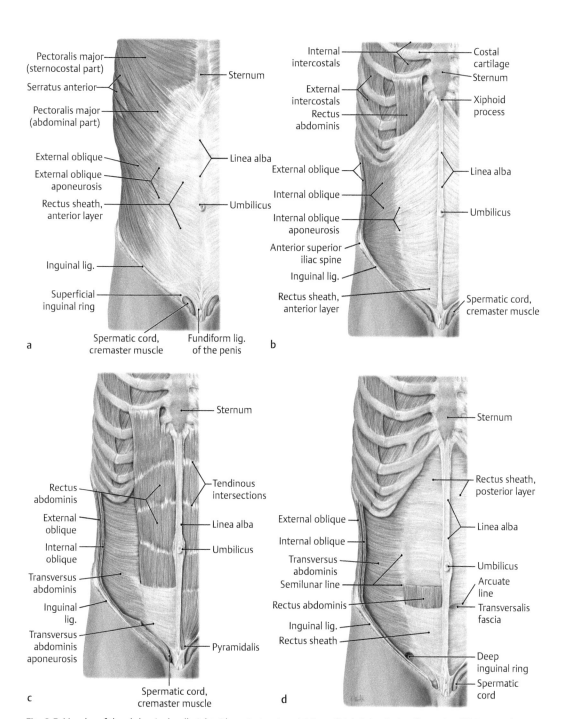

Fig. 9.5 Muscles of the abdominal wall, right side, anterior view. (**a**) Superficial abdominal wall muscles. (**b**) Removed: External oblique, pectoralis major, and serratus anterior. (**c**) Removed: Internal oblique. (**d**) Removed: Rectus abdominis. Source: From Schuenke M, Schulte E, Schumacher U. THIEME Atlas of Anatomy. General Anatomy and Musculoskeletal System. Illustrations by Voll M and Wesker K. 2nd ed. New York: Thieme Medical Publishers; 2014.

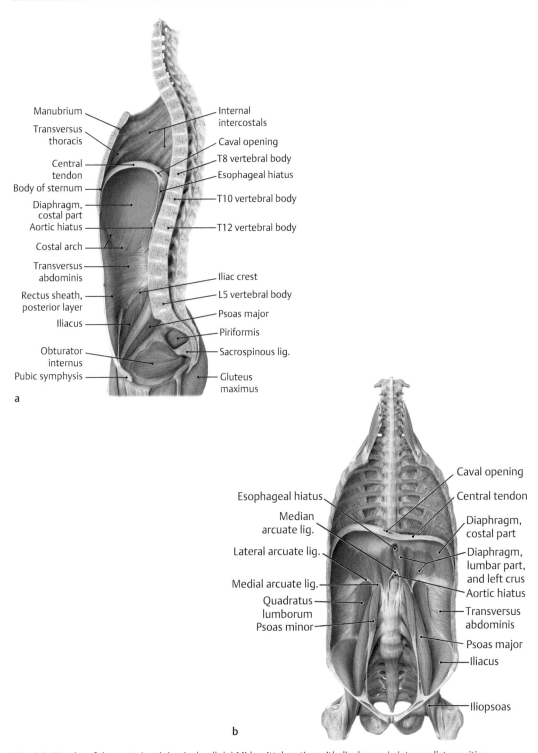

Fig. 9.6 Muscles of the posterior abdominal wall. (**a**) Midsagittal section with diaphragm in intermediate position.
(**b**) Coronal section with diaphragm in intermediate position. Source: From Schuenke M, Schulte E, Schumacher U. THIEME
Atlas of Anatomy. General Anatomy and Musculoskeletal System. Illustrations by Voll M and Wesker K. 2nd ed. New York:
Thieme Medical Publishers; 2014.

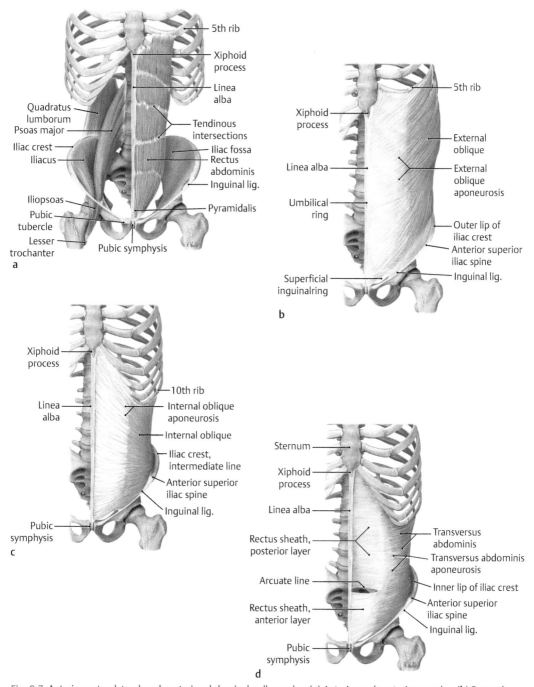

Fig. 9.7 Anterior, anterolateral, and posterior abdominal wall muscles. (**a**) Anterior and posterior muscles. (**b**) External oblique. (**c**) Internal oblique. (**d**) Transversus abdominis. Source: From Schuenke M, Schulte E, Schumacher U. THIEME Atlas of Anatomy. General Anatomy and Musculoskeletal System. Illustrations by Voll M and Wesker K. 2nd ed. New York: Thieme Medical Publishers; 2014.

Table 9.4 Abdominal wall muscles

Muscle		Origin	Insertion	Innervation	Action
Anterior abdominal wall muscles					
Rectus abdominis		*Lateral head:* Crest of pubis to pubic tubercle *Medial head:* Anterior region of pubic symphysis	Cartilages of 5th to 7th ribs, xiphoid process of sternum	Intercostal nn. (T5–T11), subcostal n. (T12)	Flexes trunk, compresses abdomen, stabilizes pelvis
Pyramidalis		Pubis (anterior to rectus abdominis)	Linea alba (runs within the rectus sheath)	Subcostal n. (T12)	Tenses linea alba
Anterolateral abdominal wall muscles					
External oblique		5th to 12th ribs (outer surface)	Linea alba, pubic tubercle, anterior iliac crest	Intercostal nn. (T7–T11), subcostal n. (T12)	*Unilateral:* Bends trunk to same side, rotates trunk to opposite side
Internal oblique		Thoracolumbar fascia (deep layer), iliac crest (intermediate line), anterior superior iliac spine, iliopsoas fascia	10th to 12th ribs (lower borders), linea alba (anterior and posterior layers)	Intercostal nn. (T7–T11), subcostal n. (T12) iliohypogastric n., ilioinguinal n.	*Bilateral:* Flexes trunk, compresses abdomen, stabilizes pelvis
Transversus abdominis		7th to 12th costal cartilages (inner surfaces), thoracolumbar fascia (deep layer), iliac crest, anterior superior iliac spine (inner lip), iliopsoas fascia	Linea alba, pubic crest		*Unilateral:* Rotates trunk to same side *Bilateral:* Compresses abdomen
Posterior abdominal wall muscles					
Psoas minor*		T12, L1 vertebrae and intervertebral disk (lateral surfaces)	Pectineal line, iliopubic ramus, iliac fascia; lowermost fibers may reach inguinal lig.		Weak flexor of the trunk
Psoas major	Superficial layer	T12–L4 vertebral bodies and associated intervertebral disks (lateral surfaces)	Femur (lesser trochanter), joint insertion as iliopsoas muscle	L1–L2 (L3) spinal nn.	*Hip joint:* Flexion and external rotation Lumbar spine (with femur fixed): *Unilateral:* Contraction bends trunk laterally *Bilateral:* Contraction raises trunk from supine position
	Deep layer	L1–L5 (costal processes)			
Iliacus		Iliac fossa		Femoral n. (L2–L4)	
Quadratus lumborum		Iliac crest and iliolumbar lig. (not shown)	12th rib, L1–L4 vertebrae (costal processes)	Subcostal n. (T12), L1–L4 spinal nn.	*Unilateral:* Bends trunk to same side *Bilateral:* Bearing down and expiration, stabilizes 12th rib

* Approximately 50% of the population has this muscle.

Source: From Gilroy AM et al. Atlas of Anatomy. 3rd ed. 2016. Based on: Schuenke M, Schulte E, Schumacher U. THIEME Atlas of Anatomy. General Anatomy and Musculoskeletal System. Illustrations by Voll M and Wesker K. 2nd ed. New York: Thieme Medical Publishers; 2014.

10 Upper Limb

Muscles of the Shoulder and Arm

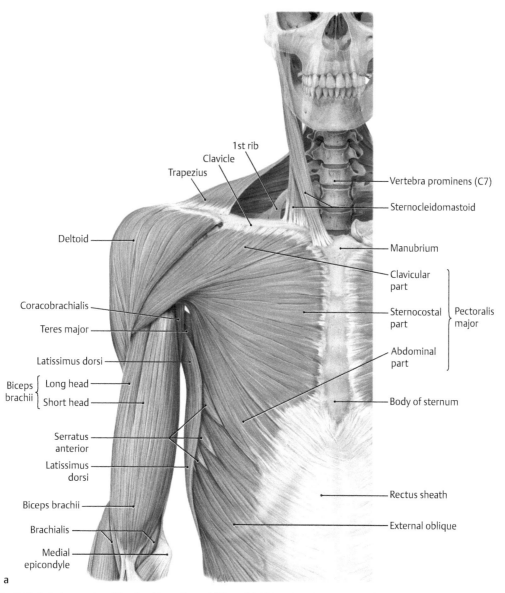

Fig. 10.1 Anterior muscles of the shoulder and arm. (**a**) Superficial dissection. Source: From Schuenke M, Schulte E, Schumacher U. THIEME Atlas of Anatomy. General Anatomy and Musculoskeletal System. Illustrations by Voll M and Wesker K. 2nd ed. New York: Thieme Medical Publishers; 2014.

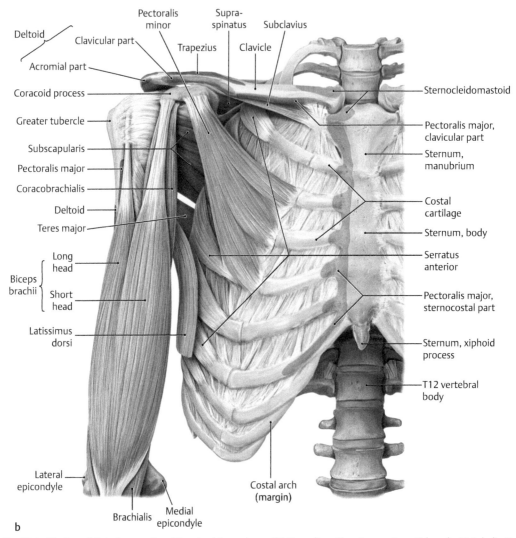

Fig. 10.1 (*Continued*) Anterior muscles of the shoulder and arm. (**b**) Deep dissection. Source: From Schuenke M, Schulte E, Schumacher U. THIEME Atlas of Anatomy. General Anatomy and Musculoskeletal System. Illustrations by Voll M and Wesker K. 2nd ed. New York: Thieme Medical Publishers; 2014.

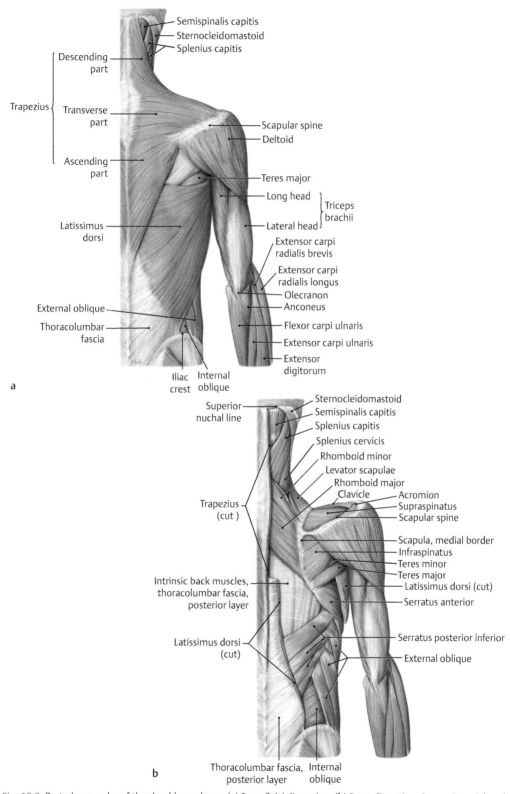

Fig. 10.2 Posterior muscles of the shoulder and arm. (**a**) Superficial dissection. (**b**) Deep dissection. Source: From Schuenke M, Schulte E, Schumacher U. THIEME Atlas of Anatomy. General Anatomy and Musculoskeletal System. Illustrations by Voll M and Wesker K. 2nd ed. New York: Thieme Medical Publishers; 2014.

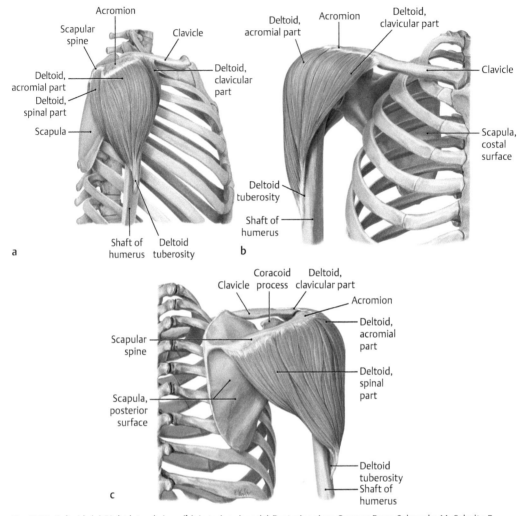

Fig. 10.3 Deltoid. (**a**) Right lateral view. (**b**) Anterior view. (**c**) Posterior view. Source: From Schuenke M, Schulte E, Schumacher U. THIEME Atlas of Anatomy. General Anatomy and Musculoskeletal System. Illustrations by Voll M and Wesker K. 2nd ed. New York: Thieme Medical Publishers; 2014.

Table 10.1 Parts of the deltoid

Muscle		Origin	Insertion	Innervation	Action*
Deltoid	Clavicular part	Lateral one third of clavicle	Humerus (deltoid tuberosity)	Axillary n. (C5, C6)	Flexion, internal rotation, adduction
	Acromial part	Acromion			Abduction
	Spinal part	Scapular spine			Extension, external rotation, adduction

* Between 60 and 90 degrees of abduction, the clavicular and spinal parts assist the acromial part with abduction.

Source: From Gilroy AM et al. Atlas of Anatomy. 3rd ed. 2016. Based on: Schuenke M, Schulte E, Schumacher U. THIEME Atlas of Anatomy. General Anatomy and Musculoskeletal System. Illustrations by Voll M and Wesker K. 2nd ed. New York: Thieme Medical Publishers; 2014.

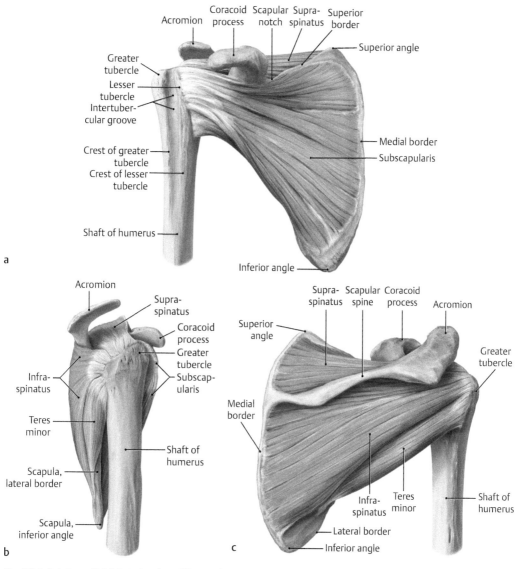

Fig. 10.4 Rotator cuff. (**a**) Anterior view. (**b**) Lateral view. (**c**) Posterior view. Source: From Schuenke M, Schulte E, Schumacher U. THIEME Atlas of Anatomy. General Anatomy and Musculoskeletal System. Illustrations by Voll M and Wesker K. 2nd ed. New York: Thieme Medical Publishers; 2014.

Table 10.2 Muscles of the rotator cuff

Muscle	Origin		Insertion		Innervation	Action
Supraspinatus		Supraspinous fossa			Suprascapular n. (C4–C6)	Abduction
Infraspinatus	Scapula	Infraspinous fossa	Humerus (greater tubercle)	Humerus		External rotation
Teres minor		Lateral border			Axillary n. (C5, C6)	External rotation, weak adduction
Subscapularis		Subscapular fossa	Humerus (lesser tubercle)		Subscapular n. (C5, C6)	Internal rotation

Source: From Gilroy AM et al. Atlas of Anatomy. 3rd ed. 2016. Based on: Schuenke M, Schulte E, Schumacher U. THIEME Atlas of Anatomy. General Anatomy and Musculoskeletal System. Illustrations by Voll M and Wesker K. 2nd ed. New York: Thieme Medical Publishers; 2014.

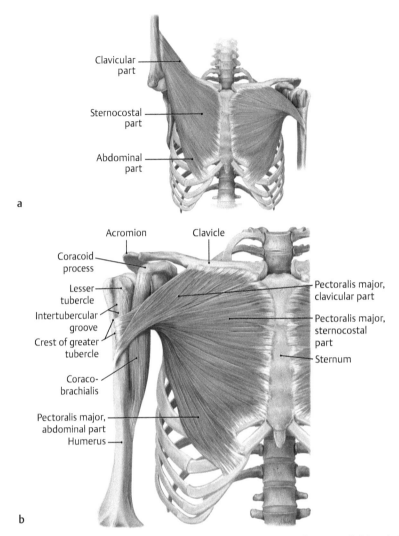

Fig. 10.5 Pectoralis major and coracobrachialis. (**a**) Pectoralis major in neutral position (left) and elevation (right). (**b**) Pectoralis major and coracobrachialis. Source: From Schuenke M, Schulte E, Schumacher U. THIEME Atlas of Anatomy. General Anatomy and Musculoskeletal System. Illustrations by Voll M and Wesker K. 2nd ed. New York: Thieme Medical Publishers; 2014.

Table 10.3 Pectoralis major and coracobrachialis

Muscle		Origin	Insertion	Innervation	Action
Pectoralis major	Clavicular part	Clavicle (medial half)	Humerus (crest of greater tubercle)	Medial and lateral pectoral nn. (C5–T1)	Entire muscle: adduction, internal rotation Clavicular and sternocostal parts: flexion; assist in respiration when shoulder is fixed
	Sternocostal part	Sternum and costal cartilages 1–6			
	Abdominal part	Rectus sheath (anterior layer)			
Coracobrachialis		Scapula (coracoid process)	Humerus (in line with crest of lesser tubercle)	Musculocutaneous n. (C5–C7)	Flexion, adduction, internal rotation

Source: From Gilroy AM et al. Atlas of Anatomy. 3rd ed. 2016. Based on: Schuenke M, Schulte E, Schumacher U. THIEME Atlas of Anatomy. General Anatomy and Musculoskeletal System. Illustrations by Voll M and Wesker K. 2nd ed. New York: Thieme Medical Publishers; 2014.

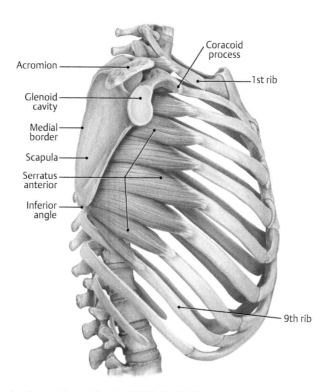

Fig. 10.6 Serratus anterior. Source: From Schuenke M, Schulte E, Schumacher U. THIEME Atlas of Anatomy. General Anatomy and Musculoskeletal System. Illustrations by Voll M and Wesker K. 2nd ed. New York: Thieme Medical Publishers; 2014.

Table 10.4 Subclavius, pectoralis minor, and serratus anterior

Muscle		Origin	Insertion	Innervation	Action
Subclavius		1st rib	Clavicle (inferior surface)	N. to subclavius (C5, C6)	Steadies the clavicle in the sternoclavicular joint
Pectoralis minor		3rd to 5th ribs	Coracoid process	Medial pectoral n. (C8, T1)	Draws scapula downward, causing inferior angle to move posteromedially; rotates glenoid inferiorly; assists in respiration
Serratus anterior	Superior part	1st to 9th ribs	Scapula (costal and dorsal surfaces of superior angle)	Long thoracic n. (C5–C7)	Superior part: lowers the raised arm
	Intermediate part		Scapula (costal surface of medial border)		Entire muscle: draws scapula laterally forward; elevates ribs when shoulder is fixed
	Inferior part		Scapula (costal surface of medial border and costal and dorsal surfaces of inferior angle)		Inferior part: rotates inferior angle of scapula laterally forward (allows elevation of arm above 90°)

Source: From Gilroy AM et al. Atlas of Anatomy. 3rd ed. 2016. Based on: Schuenke M, Schulte E, Schumacher U. THIEME Atlas of Anatomy. General Anatomy and Musculoskeletal System. Illustrations by Voll M and Wesker K. 2nd ed. New York: Thieme Medical Publishers; 2014.

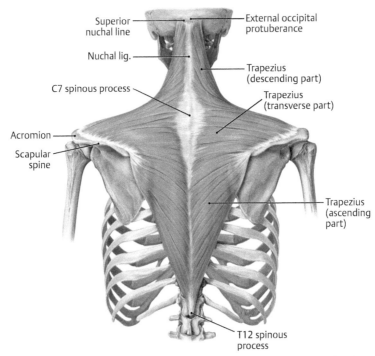

Fig. 10.7 Trapezius, posterior view. Source: From Schuenke M, Schulte E, Schumacher U. THIEME Atlas of Anatomy. General Anatomy and Musculoskeletal System. Illustrations by Voll M and Wesker K. 2nd ed. New York: Thieme Medical Publishers; 2014.

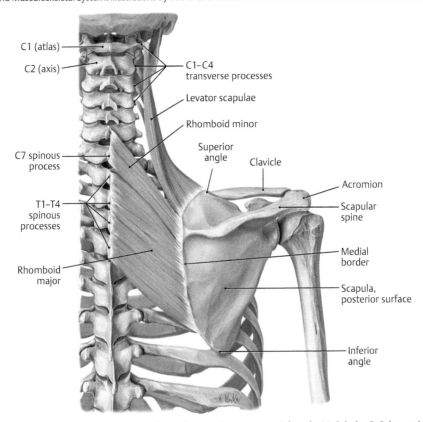

Fig. 10.8 Levator scapulae with rhomboids major and minor. Source: From Schuenke M, Schulte E, Schumacher U. THIEME Atlas of Anatomy. General Anatomy and Musculoskeletal System. Illustrations by Voll M and Wesker K. 2nd ed. New York: Thieme Medical Publishers; 2014.

Table 10.5 Trapezius, levator scapulae, and rhomboids major and minor

Muscle		Origin	Insertion	Innervation	Action
Trapezius	Descending part	Occipital bone; spinous processes of C1–C7	Clavicle (lateral one third)	Accessory n. (CN XI); C3–C4 of cervical plexus	Draws scapula obliquely upward; rotates glenoid cavity superiorly; tilts head to same side and rotates it to opposite
	Transverse part	Aponeurosis at T1–T4 spinous processes	Acromion		Draws scapula medially
	Ascending part	Spinous processes of T5–T12	Scapular spine		Draws scapula medially downward
					Entire muscle: steadies scapula on thorax
Levator scapulae		Transverse processes of C1–C4	Scapula (superior angle)	Dorsal scapular n. and cervical spinal nn. (C3–C4)	Draws scapula medially upward while moving inferior angle medially; inclines neck to same side
Rhomboid minor		Spinous processes of C6, C7	Medial border of scapula above (minor) and below (major) scapular spine	Dorsal scapular n. (C4–C5)	Steadies scapula; draws scapula medially upward
Rhomboid major		Spinous processes of T1–T4 vertebrae			

Abbreviation: CN, cranial nerve.

Source: From Gilroy AM et al. Atlas of Anatomy. 3rd ed. 2016. Based on: Schuenke M, Schulte E, Schumacher U. THIEME Atlas of Anatomy. General Anatomy and Musculoskeletal System. Illustrations by Voll M and Wesker K. 2nd ed. New York: Thieme Medical Publishers; 2014.

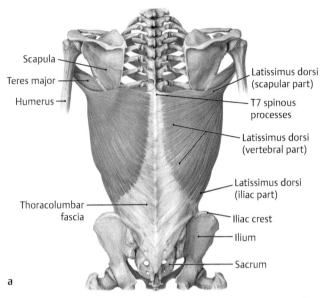

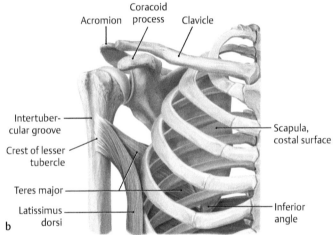

Fig. 10.9 (**a**) Latissimus dorsi and teres major. (**b**) Insertion of the latissimus dorsi on the floor of the intertubercular groove and the teres major on the crest of the lesser tubercle of the humerus. Source: From Schuenke M, Schulte E, Schumacher U. THIEME Atlas of Anatomy. General Anatomy and Musculoskeletal System. Illustrations by Voll M and Wesker K. 2nd ed. New York: Thieme Medical Publishers; 2014.

Table 10.6 Latissimus dorsi and teres major

Muscle		Origin	Insertion	Innervation	Action
Latissimus dorsi	Vertebral part	Spinous processes of T7–T12 vertebrae; thoracolumbar fascia	Floor of the intertubercular groove of the humerus	Thoracodorsal n. (C6–C8)	Internal rotation, adduction, extension, respiration ("cough muscle")
	Scapular part	Scapula (inferior angle)			
	Costal part	9th to 12th ribs			
	Iliac part	Iliac crest (posterior one third)			
Teres major		Scapula (inferior angle)	Crest of lesser tubercle of the humerus (anterior angle)	Lower subscapular n. (C5–C7)	Internal rotation, adduction, extension

Source: From Gilroy AM et al. Atlas of Anatomy. 3rd ed. 2016. Based on: Schuenke M, Schulte E, Schumacher U. THIEME Atlas of Anatomy. General Anatomy and Musculoskeletal System. Illustrations by Voll M and Wesker K. 2nd ed. New York: Thieme Medical Publishers; 2014.

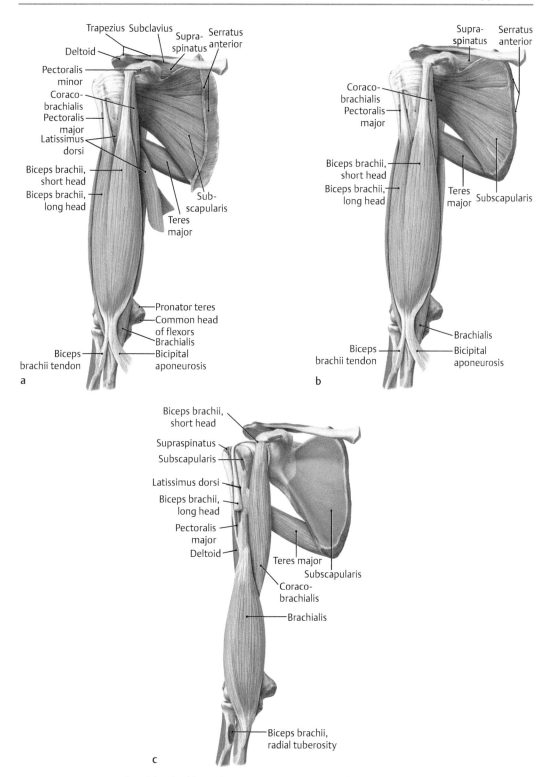

Fig. 10.10 Anterior muscles of the shoulder and arm: Dissection. (**a**) Removed: Thoracic skeleton. Partially removed: Latissimus dorsi and serratus anterior. (**b**) Removed: Latissimus dorsi and serratus anterior. (**c**) Removed: Subscapularis and supraspinatus. Partially removed: Biceps brachii. Source: From Schuenke M, Schulte E, Schumacher U. THIEME Atlas of Anatomy. General Anatomy and Musculoskeletal System. Illustrations by Voll M and Wesker K. 2nd ed. New York: Thieme Medical Publishers; 2014.

Table 10.7 Anterior muscles: biceps brachii and brachialis

Muscle		Origin	Insertion	Innervation	Action
Biceps brachii	Long head	Supraglenoid tubercle of scapula			Elbow joint: flexion; supination*
	Short head	Coracoid process of scapula	Radial tuberosity and bicipital aponeurosis	Musculocutaneous n. (C5–C6)	Shoulder joint: flexion; stabilization of humeral head during deltoid contraction; abduction and internal rotation of the humerus
Brachialis		Humerus (distal half of anterior surface)	Ulnar tuberosity	Musculocutaneous n. (C5–C6) and radial n. (C7, minor)	Flexion at the elbow joint

*Note: When the elbow is flexed, the biceps brachii acts as a powerful supinator because the lever arm is almost perpendicular to the axis of pronation/supination.

Source: From Gilroy AM et al. Atlas of Anatomy. 3rd ed. 2016. Based on: Schuenke M, Schulte E, Schumacher U. THIEME Atlas of Anatomy. General Anatomy and Musculoskeletal System. Illustrations by Voll M and Wesker K. 2nd ed. New York: Thieme Medical Publishers; 2014.

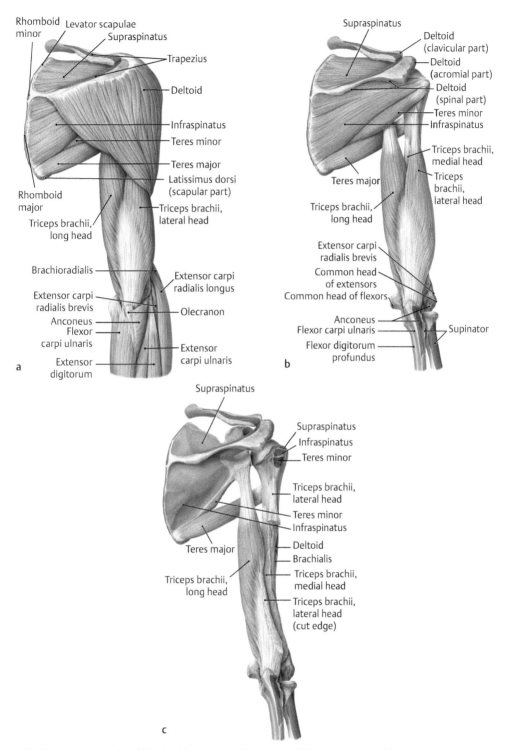

Fig. 10.11 Posterior muscles of the shoulder and arm: Dissection. (**a**) Removed: Rhomboids major and minor, serratus anterior, and levator scapulae. (**b**) Removed: Deltoid and forearm muscles. (**c**) Removed: Supraspinatus, infraspinatus, and teres minor. Partially removed: Triceps brachii. Source: From Schuenke M, Schulte E, Schumacher U. THIEME Atlas of Anatomy. General Anatomy and Musculoskeletal System. Illustrations by Voll M and Wesker K. 2nd ed. New York: Thieme Medical Publishers; 2014.

Table 10.8 Posterior muscles: triceps brachii and anconeus

Muscle		Origin	Insertion	Innervation	Action
Triceps brachii	Long head	Scapula (infraglenoid tubercle)	Olecranon of ulna	Radial n. (C6–C8)	Elbow joint: extension Shoulder joint, long head: extension and adduction
	Medial head	Posterior humerus, distal to radial groove; medial intermuscular septum			
	Lateral head	Posterior humerus, proximal to radial groove; lateral intermuscular septum			
Anconeus		Lateral epicondyle of humerus (variance: posterior joint capsule)	Olecranon of ulna (radial surface)		Extends the elbow and tightens its joint

Source: From Gilroy AM et al. Atlas of Anatomy. 3rd ed. 2016. Based on: Schuenke M, Schulte E, Schumacher U. THIEME Atlas of Anatomy. General Anatomy and Musculoskeletal System. Illustrations by Voll M and Wesker K. 2nd ed. New York: Thieme Medical Publishers; 2014.

Muscles of the Forearm and Hand

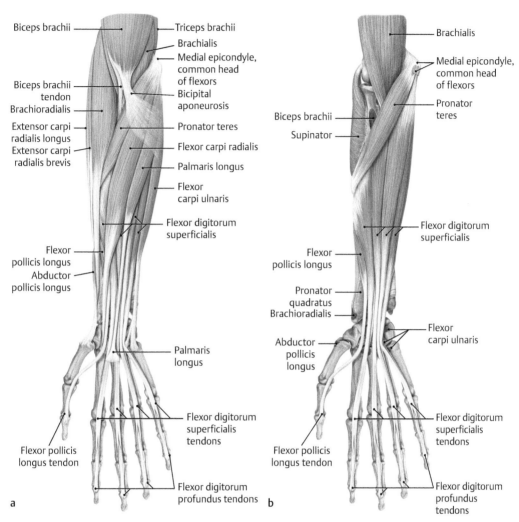

Biceps brachii

Triceps brachii

Brachialis

Medial epicondyle, common head of flexors

Biceps brachii tendon

Bicipital aponeurosis

Brachioradialis

Pronator teres

Extensor carpi radialis longus

Flexor carpi radialis

Extensor carpi radialis brevis

Palmaris longus

Flexor carpi ulnaris

Flexor digitorum superficialis

Flexor pollicis longus

Abductor pollicis longus

Palmaris longus

Flexor digitorum superficialis tendons

Flexor pollicis longus tendon

Flexor digitorum profundus tendons

a

Brachialis

Medial epicondyle, common head of flexors

Pronator teres

Biceps brachii

Supinator

Flexor digitorum superficialis

Flexor pollicis longus

Pronator quadratus

Brachioradialis

Flexor carpi ulnaris

Abductor pollicis longus

Flexor digitorum superficialis tendons

Flexor pollicis longus tendon

Flexor digitorum profundus tendons

b

Fig. 10.12 Anterior muscles of the forearm: Dissection. (**a**) Superficial flexors and radialis muscles. (**b**) Removed: Radialis muscles (brachioradialis, extensor carpi radialis longus, and extensor carpi radialis brevis), flexor carpi radialis, flexor carpi ulnaris, abductor pollicis longus, palmaris longus, and biceps brachii. Source: From Schuenke M, Schulte E, Schumacher U. THIEME Atlas of Anatomy. General Anatomy and Musculoskeletal System. Illustrations by Voll M and Wesker K. 2nd ed. New York: Thieme Medical Publishers; 2014.

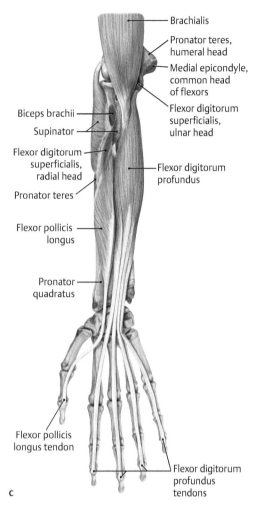

Brachialis

Pronator teres, humeral head

Medial epicondyle, common head of flexors

Flexor digitorum superficialis, ulnar head

Biceps brachii

Supinator

Flexor digitorum superficialis, radial head

Pronator teres

Flexor digitorum profundus

Flexor pollicis longus

Pronator quadratus

Flexor pollicis longus tendon

Flexor digitorum profundus tendons

c

Fig. 10.12 (*Continued*) Anterior muscles of the forearm: Dissection. (**c**) Removed: Pronator teres and flexor digitorum superficialis. Source: From Schuenke M, Schulte E, Schumacher U. THIEME Atlas of Anatomy. General Anatomy and Musculoskeletal System. Illustrations by Voll M and Wesker K. 2nd ed. New York: Thieme Medical Publishers; 2014.

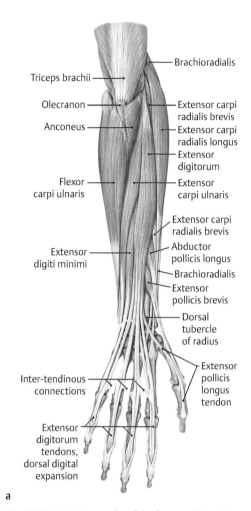

Brachioradialis

Triceps brachii

Olecranon

Anconeus

Extensor carpi radialis brevis

Extensor carpi radialis longus

Extensor digitorum

Flexor carpi ulnaris

Extensor carpi ulnaris

Extensor carpi radialis brevis

Abductor pollicis longus

Extensor digiti minimi

Brachioradialis

Extensor pollicis brevis

Dorsal tubercle of radius

Extensor pollicis longus tendon

Inter-tendinous connections

Extensor digitorum tendons, dorsal digital expansion

a

Fig. 10.13 Posterior muscles of the forearm: Dissection. (**a**) Superficial extensors and radialis group. Source: From Schuenke M, Schulte E, Schumacher U. THIEME Atlas of Anatomy. General Anatomy and Musculoskeletal System. Illustrations by Voll M and Wesker K. 2nd ed. New York: Thieme Medical Publishers; 2014.

Table 10.9 Anterior compartment of the forearm

Muscle	Origin	Insertion	Innervation	Action
Superficial muscles				
Pronator teres	Humeral head: medial epicondyle of humerus Ulnar head: coronoid process	Lateral radius (distal to supinator insertion)	Median n. (C6, C7)	Elbow: weak flexion Forearm: pronation
Flexor carpi radialis	Medial epicondyle of humerus	Base of 2nd metacarpal (variance: base of 3rd metacarpal)		Wrist: flexion and abduction (radial deviation) of hand
Palmaris longus		Palmar aponeurosis	Median n. (C7, C8)	Elbow: weak flexion Wrist: flexion tightens palmar aponeurosis
Flexor carpi ulnaris	Humeral head: medial epicondyle Ulnar head: olecranon	Pisiform; hook of hamate; base of 5th metacarpal	Ulnar n. (C7–T1)	Wrist: flexion and adduction (ulnar deviation) of hand
Intermediate muscles				
Flexor digitorum superficialis	Humeral-ulnar head: medial epicondyle of humerus and coronoid process of ulna Radial head: upper half of anterior border of radius	Sides of middle phalanges of 2nd to 5th digits	Median n. (C8, T1)	Elbow: weak flexion Wrist, MCP, and PIP joints of 2nd to 5th digits: flexion
Deep muscles				
Flexor digitorum profundus	Ulna (proximal two thirds of flexor surface) and interosseous membrane	Distal phalanges of 2nd to 5th digits (palmar surface)	Median n. (C8, T1, radial half of fingers 2 and 3) Ulnar n. (C8, T1, ulnar half of fingers 4 and 5)	Wrist, MCP, PIP, and DIP joints of 2nd to 5th digits: flexion
Flexor pollicis longus	Radius (midanterior surface) and adjacent interosseous membrane	Distal phalanx of thumb (palmar surface)	Median n. (C8, T1)	Wrist: flexion and abduction (radial deviation) of hand Carpometacarpal joint of thumb: flexion MCP and IP joints of thumb: flexion
Pronator qua-dratus	Distal quarter of ulna (anterior surface)	Distal quarter of radius (anterior surface)		Hand: pronation Distal radioulnar joint: stabilization

Abbreviations: DIP, distal interphalangeal; IP, interphalangeal; MCP, metacarpophalangeal; PIP, proximal interphalangeal.
Source: From Gilroy AM et al. Atlas of Anatomy. 3rd ed. 2016. Based on: Schuenke M, Schulte E, Schumacher U. THIEME Atlas of Anatomy. General Anatomy and Musculoskeletal System. Illustrations by Voll M and Wesker K. 2nd ed. New York: Thieme Medical Publishers; 2014.

Table 10.10 Posterior compartment of the forearm: radialis muscles

Muscle	Origin	Insertion	Innervation	Action
Brachioradialis	Distal humerus (lateral surface), lateral intermuscular septum	Styloid process of the radius	Radial n. (C5, C6)	Elbow: flexion Forearm: semipronation
Extensor carpi radialis longus	Lateral supracondylar ridge of distal humerus, lateral intermuscular septum	2nd metacarpal (base)	Radial n. (C6, C7)	Elbow: weak flexion Wrist: extension and abduction
Extensor carpi radialis brevis	Lateral epicondyle of humerus	3rd metacarpal (base)	Radial n. (C7, C8)	

Source: From Gilroy AM et al. Atlas of Anatomy. 3rd ed. 2016. Based on: Schuenke M, Schulte E, Schumacher U. THIEME Atlas of Anatomy. General Anatomy and Musculoskeletal System. Illustrations by Voll M and Wesker K. 2nd ed. New York: Thieme Medical Publishers; 2014.

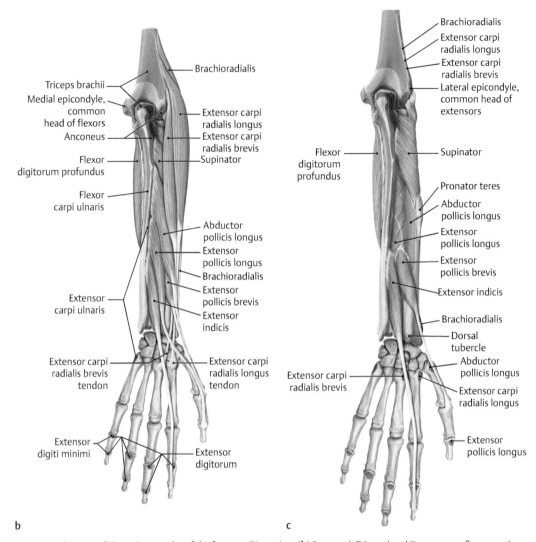

Brachioradialis

Triceps brachii
Medial epicondyle, common head of flexors
Anconeus
Flexor digitorum profundus
Flexor carpi ulnaris

Extensor carpi radialis longus
Extensor carpi radialis brevis
Supinator

Abductor pollicis longus
Extensor pollicis longus
Brachioradialis
Extensor pollicis brevis
Extensor indicis

Extensor carpi ulnaris

Extensor carpi radialis brevis tendon

Extensor carpi radialis longus tendon

Extensor digiti minimi

Extensor digitorum

b

Brachioradialis
Extensor carpi radialis longus
Extensor carpi radialis brevis
Lateral epicondyle, common head of extensors

Flexor digitorum profundus

Supinator

Pronator teres
Abductor pollicis longus
Extensor pollicis longus
Extensor pollicis brevis
Extensor indicis

Brachioradialis
Dorsal tubercle
Abductor pollicis longus
Extensor carpi radialis longus

Extensor carpi radialis brevis

Extensor pollicis longus

c

Fig. 10.13 (*Continued*) Posterior muscles of the forearm: Dissection. (**b**) Removed: Triceps brachii, anconeus, flexor carpi ulnaris, extensor carpi ulnaris, and extensor digitorum. (**c**) Removed: Abductor pollicis longus, extensor pollicis longus, and radialis muscles. Source: From Schuenke M, Schulte E, Schumacher U. THIEME Atlas of Anatomy. General Anatomy and Musculoskeletal System. Illustrations by Voll M and Wesker K. 2nd ed. New York: Thieme Medical Publishers; 2014.

Table 10.11 Posterior compartment of the forearm

Muscle	Origin	Insertion	Innervation	Action
Superficial muscles				
Extensor digitorum	Common head (lateral epicondyle of humerus)	Dorsal digital expansion of 2nd to 5th digits	Radial n. (C7, C8)	Wrist: extension MCP, PIP, and DIP joints of 2nd to 5th digits: extension/abduction of fingers
Extensor digiti minimi		Dorsal digital expansion of 5th digit		Wrist: extension, ulnar abduction of hand MCP, PIP, and DIP joints of 5th digit: extension and abduction of 5th digit
Extensor carpi ulnaris	Common head (lateral epicondyle of humerus) Ulnar head (dorsal surface)	Base of 5th metacarpal		Wrist: extension, adduction (ulnar deviation) of hand
Deep muscles				
Supinator	Olecranon, lateral epicondyle of humerus, radial collateral ligament, annular ligament of radius	Radius (between radial tuberosity and insertion of pronator teres)	Radial n. (C6, C7)	Radioulnar joints: supination
Abductor pollicis longus	Radius and ulna (dorsal surfaces, interosseous membrane)	Base of 1st metacarpal	Radial n. (C7, C8)	Radiocarpal joint: abduction of the hand Carpometacarpal joint of thumb: abduction
Extensor pollicis brevis	Radius (posterior surface) and interosseous membrane	Base of proximal phalanx of thumb		Radiocarpal joint: abduction (radial deviation) of hand Carpometacarpal and MCP joints of thumb: extension
Extensor pollicis longus	Ulna (posterior surface) and interosseous membrane	Base of distal phalanx of thumb		Wrist: extension and abduction (radial deviation) of hand Carpometacarpal joint of thumb: adduction MCP and IP joints of thumb: extension
Extensor indicis	Ulna (posterior surface) and interosseous membrane	Posterior digital extension of 2nd digit		Wrist: extension MCP, PIP, and DIP joints of 2nd digit: extension

Abbreviations: DIP, distal interphalangeal; IP, interphalangeal; MCP, metacarpophalangeal; PIP, proximal interphalangeal.

Source: From Gilroy AM et al. Atlas of Anatomy. 3rd ed. 2016. Based on: Schuenke M, Schulte E, Schumacher U. THIEME Atlas of Anatomy. General Anatomy and Musculoskeletal System. Illustrations by Voll M and Wesker K. 2nd ed. New York: Thieme Medical Publishers; 2014.

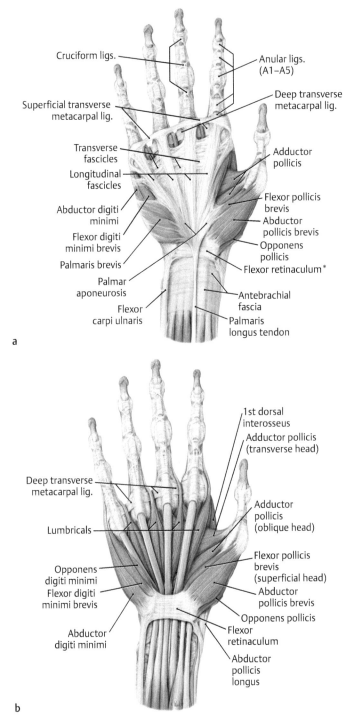

Cruciform ligs.

Anular ligs.
(A1–A5)

Superficial transverse
metacarpal lig.

Deep transverse
metacarpal lig.

Transverse
fascicles

Adductor
pollicis

Longitudinal
fascicles

Abductor digiti
minimi

Flexor pollicis
brevis

Abductor
pollicis brevis

Flexor digiti
minimi brevis

Opponens
pollicis

Palmaris brevis

Flexor retinaculum*

Palmar
aponeurosis

Antebrachial
fascia

Flexor
carpi ulnaris

Palmaris
longus tendon

a

1st dorsal
interosseus

Adductor pollicis
(transverse head)

Deep transverse
metacarpal lig.

Adductor
pollicis
(oblique head)

Lumbricals

Flexor pollicis
brevis
(superficial head)

Opponens
digiti minimi

Abductor
pollicis brevis

Flexor digiti
minimi brevis

Opponens pollicis

Flexor
retinaculum

Abductor
digiti minimi

Abductor
pollicis
longus

b

Fig. 10.14 Intrinsic muscles of the hand: superficial and middle layers. (**a**) Palmar aponeurosis. (*also known as transverse carpal ligament.) (**b**) Superficial layer of muscles. Source: From Schuenke M, Schulte E, Schumacher U. THIEME Atlas of Anatomy. General Anatomy and Musculoskeletal System. Illustrations by Voll M and Wesker K. 2nd ed. New York: Thieme Medical Publishers; 2014.

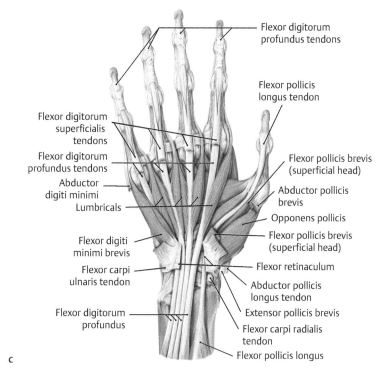

Flexor digitorum
profundus tendons

Flexor pollicis
longus tendon

Flexor digitorum
superficialis
tendons

Flexor digitorum
profundus tendons

Abductor
digiti minimi

Lumbricals

Flexor digiti
minimi brevis

Flexor carpi
ulnaris tendon

Flexor digitorum
profundus

Flexor pollicis brevis
(superficial head)

Abductor pollicis
brevis

Opponens pollicis

Flexor pollicis brevis
(superficial head)

Flexor retinaculum

Abductor pollicis
longus tendon

Extensor pollicis brevis

Flexor carpi radialis
tendon

Flexor pollicis longus

c

Fig. 10.14 (*Continued*) Intrinsic muscles of the hand: superficial and middle layers. (**c**) Middle layer of muscles. Source: From Schuenke M, Schulte E, Schumacher U. THIEME Atlas of Anatomy. General Anatomy and Musculoskeletal System. Illustrations by Voll M and Wesker K. 2nd ed. New York: Thieme Medical Publishers; 2014.

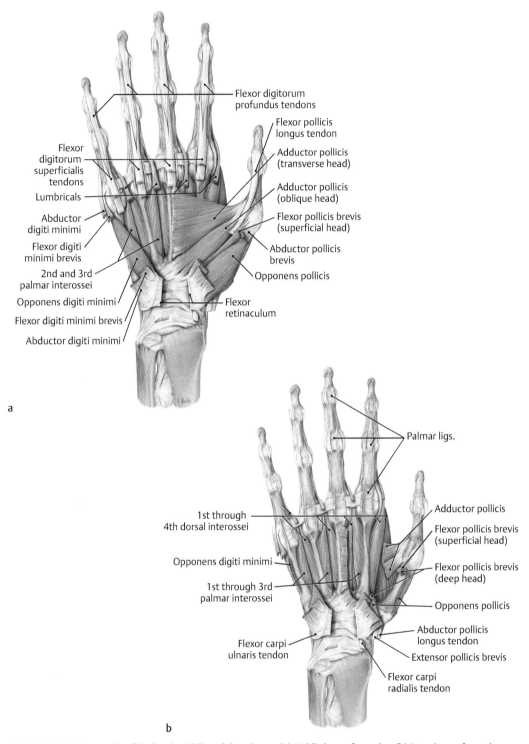

a

Flexor digitorum profundus tendons

Flexor pollicis longus tendon

Adductor pollicis (transverse head)

Adductor pollicis (oblique head)

Flexor pollicis brevis (superficial head)

Abductor pollicis brevis

Opponens pollicis

Flexor retinaculum

Flexor digitorum superficialis tendons

Lumbricals

Abductor digiti minimi

Flexor digiti minimi brevis

2nd and 3rd palmar interossei

Opponens digiti minimi

Flexor digiti minimi brevis

Abductor digiti minimi

Palmar ligs.

1st through 4th dorsal interossei

Opponens digiti minimi

1st through 3rd palmar interossei

Flexor carpi ulnaris tendon

Adductor pollicis

Flexor pollicis brevis (superficial head)

Flexor pollicis brevis (deep head)

Opponens pollicis

Abductor pollicis longus tendon

Extensor pollicis brevis

Flexor carpi radialis tendon

b

Fig. 10.15 Intrinsic muscles of the hand: middle and deep layers. (**a**) Middle layer of muscles. (**b**) Deep layer of muscles. Source: From Schuenke M, Schulte E, Schumacher U. THIEME Atlas of Anatomy. General Anatomy and Musculoskeletal System. Illustrations by Voll M and Wesker K. 2nd ed. New York: Thieme Medical Publishers; 2014.

11 Lower Limb

Muscles of the Hip and Thigh

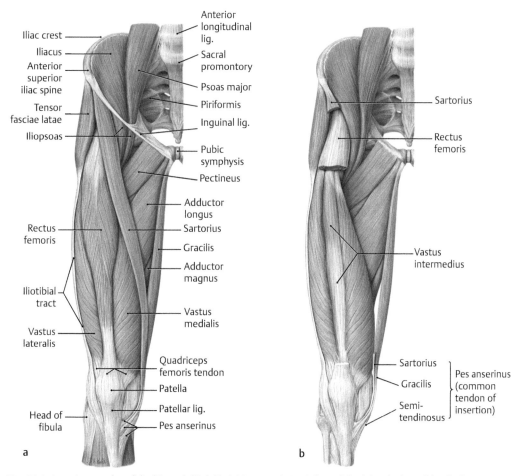

Fig. 11.1 Anterior muscles of the hip and thigh (I). (**a**) Removed: Fascia lata of thigh (to the lateral iliotibial tract). (**b**) Removed: Inguinal ligament, sartorius and rectus femoris. Source: From Schuenke M, Schulte E, Schumacher U. THIEME Atlas of Anatomy. General Anatomy and Musculoskeletal System. Illustrations by Voll M and Wesker K. 2nd ed. New York: Thieme Medical Publishers; 2014.

Table 11.1 Iliopsoas muscle

Muscle		Origin	Insertion	Innervation	Action
Iliopsoas	Psoas major*	*Superficial:* T12–L4 and associated intervertebral disks (lateral surfaces) *Deep:* L1–L5 vertebrae (costal processes)	Femur (lesser trochanter)	Lumbar plexus L1, L2(L3)	• Hip joint: flexion and external rotation • Lumbar spine: *unilateral* contraction (with the femur fixed) bends the trunk laterally to the same side; *bilateral* contraction raises the trunk from the supine position
	Iliacus	Iliac fossa		Femoral n. (L2–L3)	

* The psoas minor, present in approximately 50% of the population, is often found on the superficial surface of the psoas major. It is not a muscle of the lower limb. It originates, inserts, and exerts its action on the abdomen (see **Table 9.4**).

Source: From Gilroy AM et al. Atlas of Anatomy. 3rd ed. 2016. Based on: Schuenke M, Schulte E, Schumacher U. THIEME Atlas of Anatomy. General Anatomy and Musculoskeletal System. Illustrations by Voll M and Wesker K. 2nd ed. New York: Thieme Medical Publishers; 2014.

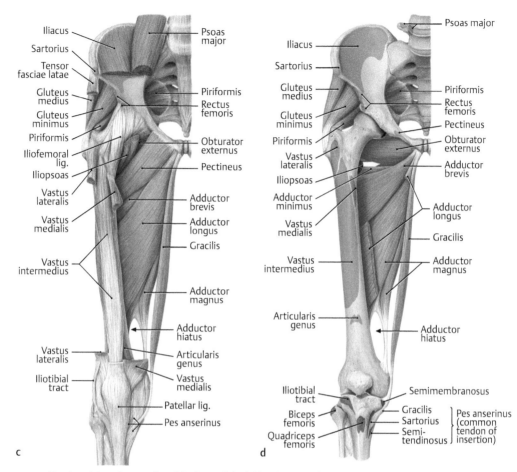

Fig. 11.1 (*Continued*) Anterior muscles of the hip and thigh (I). (**c**) Removed: Rectus femoris (completely), vastus lateralis, vastus mediais, iliopsoas, and tensor fasciae latae. (**d**) Removed: Quadriceps femoris (rectus femoris, vastus lateralis, vastus medialis, vastus intermedius), iliopsoas, tensor fasciae latae, pectineus, and midportion of adductor longus. Source: From Schuenke M, Schulte E, Schumacher U. THIEME Atlas of Anatomy. General Anatomy and Musculoskeletal System. Illustrations by Voll M and Wesker K. 2nd ed. New York: Thieme Medical Publishers; 2014.

Table 11.2 Medial thigh muscles: superficial layer

Muscle	Origin	Insertion	Innervation	Action
Pectineus	Pecten pubis	Femur (pectineal line and the proximal linea aspera)	Femoral n., obturator n. (L2, L3)	• Hip joint: adduction, external rotation, and slight flexion • Stabilizes the pelvis in the coronal and sagittal planes
Adductor longus	Superior pubic ramus and anterior side of the pubic symphysis	Femur (linea aspera, medial lip in the middle third of the femur)	Obturator n. (L2–L4)	• Hip joint: adduction and flexion (up to 70 degrees); extension (past 80 degrees of flexion) • Stabilizes the pelvis in the coronal and sagittal planes
Adductor brevis	Inferior pubic ramus			
Gracilis	Inferior pubic ramus below the pubic symphysis	Tibia (medial border of the tuberosity, along with the tendons of sartorius and semitendinosus)	Obturator n. (L2, L3)	• Hip joint: adduction and flexion • Knee joint: flexion and internal rotation

Source: From Gilroy AM et al. Atlas of Anatomy. 3rd ed. 2016. Based on: Schuenke M, Schulte E, Schumacher U. THIEME Atlas of Anatomy. General Anatomy and Musculoskeletal System. Illustrations by Voll M and Wesker K. 2nd ed. New York: Thieme Medical Publishers; 2014.

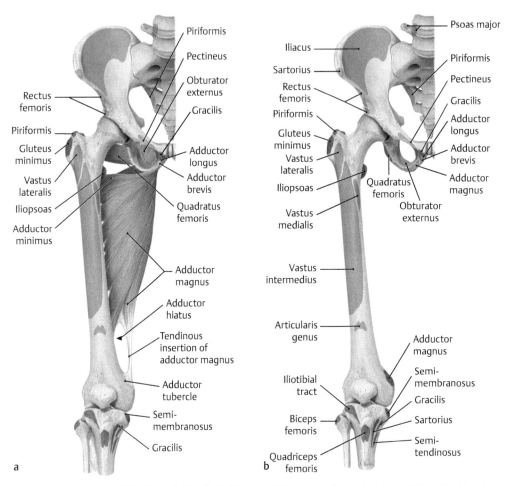

Fig. 11.2 Anterior muscles of the hip and thigh (II). (**a**) Removed: Gluteus medius and minimus, piriformis, obturator externus, adductor brevis and longus, and gracilis. (**b**) Removed: All muscles. Source: From Schuenke M, Schulte E, Schumacher U. THIEME Atlas of Anatomy. General Anatomy and Musculoskeletal System. Illustrations by Voll M and Wesker K. 2nd ed. New York: Thieme Medical Publishers; 2014.

Table 11.3 Medial thigh muscles: deep layer

Muscle	Origin	Insertion	Innervation	Action
Obturator externus	Outer surface of the obturator membrane and its bony boundaries	Trochanteric fossa of the femur	Obturator n. (L3, L4)	• Hip joint: adduction and external rotation • Stabilizes the pelvis in the sagittal plane
Adductor magnus	Inferior pubic ramus, ischial ramus, and ischial tuberosity	• Deep part ("fleshy insertion"): medial lip of the linea aspera • Superficial part ("tendinous insertion"): adductor tubercle of the femur	• Deep part: obturator n. (L2–L4) • Superficial part: tibial n. (L4)	• Hip joint: adduction, extension, and slight flexion (the tendinous insertion is also active in internal rotation) • Stabilizes the pelvis in the coronal and sagittal planes

Source: From Gilroy AM et al. Atlas of Anatomy. 3rd ed. 2016. Based on: Schuenke M, Schulte E, Schumacher U. THIEME Atlas of Anatomy. General Anatomy and Musculoskeletal System. Illustrations by Voll M and Wesker K. 2nd ed. New York: Thieme Medical Publishers; 2014.

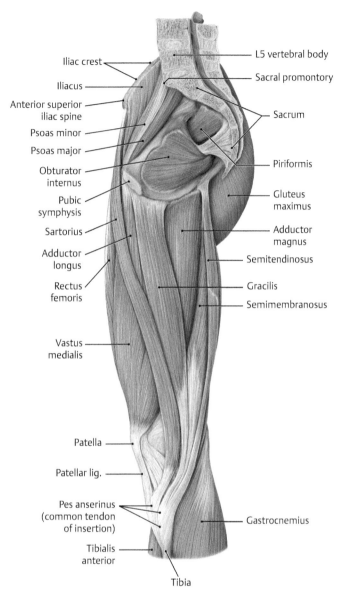

Fig. 11.3 Medial muscles of the hip, thigh, and gluteal region. Source: From Schuenke M, Schulte E, Schumacher U. THIEME Atlas of Anatomy. General Anatomy and Musculoskeletal System. Illustrations by Voll M and Wesker K. 2nd ed. New York: Thieme Medical Publishers; 2014.

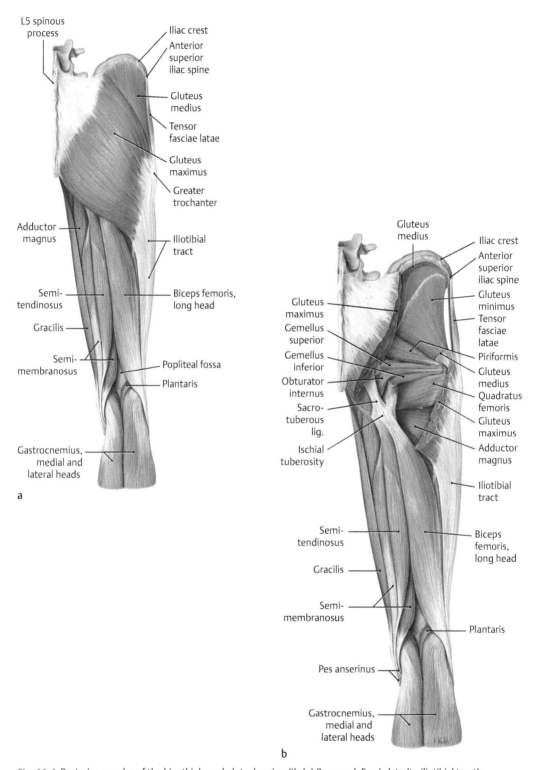

Fig. 11.4 Posterior muscles of the hip, thigh, and gluteal region (I). (**a**) Removed: Fascia lata (to iliotibial tract). (**b**) Partially removed: Gluteus maximus and medius. Source: From Schuenke M, Schulte E, Schumacher U. THIEME Atlas of Anatomy. General Anatomy and Musculoskeletal System. Illustrations by Voll M and Wesker K. 2nd ed. New York: Thieme Medical Publishers; 2014.

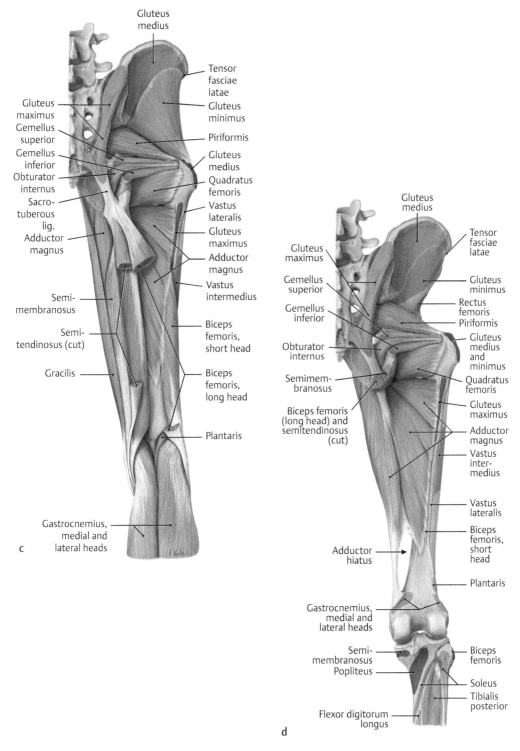

Fig. 11.4 (*Continued*) Posterior muscles of the hip, thigh, and gluteal region (I). (**c**) Removed: Semitendinosus and biceps femoris (partially); gluteus maximus and medius (completely). (**d**) Removed: Hamstrings (semitendinosus, semimembranosus, and biceps femoris), gluteus minimus, gastrocnemius, and muscles of the leg. Source: From Schuenke M, Schulte E, Schumacher U. THIEME Atlas of Anatomy. General Anatomy and Musculoskeletal System. Illustrations by Voll M and Wesker K. 2nd ed. New York: Thieme Medical Publishers; 2014.

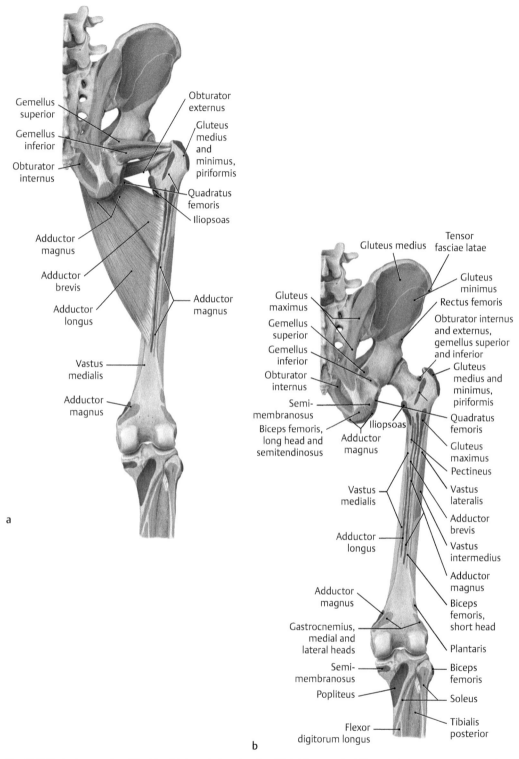

Gemellus superior

Gemellus inferior

Obturator internus

Obturator externus

Gluteus medius and minimus, piriformis

Quadratus femoris

Iliopsoas

Adductor magnus

Adductor brevis

Adductor longus

Adductor magnus

Vastus medialis

Adductor magnus

a

Tensor fasciae latae

Gluteus medius

Gluteus minimus

Rectus femoris

Obturator internus and externus, gemellus superior and inferior

Gluteus medius and minimus, piriformis

Quadratus femoris

Gluteus maximus

Pectineus

Vastus lateralis

Adductor brevis

Vastus intermedius

Adductor magnus

Biceps femoris, short head

Plantaris

Biceps femoris

Soleus

Tibialis posterior

Gluteus maximus

Gemellus superior

Gemellus inferior

Obturator internus

Semi-membranosus

Biceps femoris, long head and semitendinosus

Iliopsoas

Adductor magnus

Vastus medialis

Adductor longus

Adductor magnus

Gastrocnemius, medial and lateral heads

Semi-membranosus

Popliteus

Flexor digitorum longus

b

Fig. 11.5 Posterior muscles of the hip, thigh, and gluteal region (II). (a) Removed: Piriformis, obturator internus, quadratus femoris, and adductor magnus. (b) Removed: All muscles. Source: From Schuenke M, Schulte E, Schumacher U. THIEME Atlas of Anatomy. General Anatomy and Musculoskeletal System. Illustrations by Voll M and Wesker K. 2nd ed. New York: Thieme Medical Publishers; 2014.

Table 11.4 Gluteal muscles

Muscle	Origin	Insertion	Innervation	Action
Gluteus maximus	Sacrum (dorsal surface, lateral part), ilium (gluteal surface, posterior part), thoracolumbar fascia, sacrotuberous lig.	• Upper fibers: iliotibial tract • Lower fibers: gluteal tuberosity	Inferior gluteal n. (L5–S2)	• Entire muscle: extends and externally rotates the hip in sagittal and coronal planes • Upper fibers: abduction • Lower fibers: adduction
Gluteus medius	Ilium (gluteal surface below the iliac crest between the anterior and posterior gluteal line)	Greater trochanter of the femur (lateral surface)	Superior gluteal n. (L4–S1)	• Entire muscle: abducts the hip, stabilizes the pelvis in the coronal plane • Anterior part: flexion and internal rotation • Posterior part: extension and external rotation
Gluteus minimus	Ilium (gluteal surface below the origin of gluteus medius)	Greater trochanter of the femur (anterolateral surface)		
Tensor fasciae latae	Anterior superior iliac spine	Iliotibial tract		• Tenses the fascia lata • Hip joint: abduction, flexion, and internal rotation
Piriformis	Pelvic surface of the sacrum	Apex of the greater trochanter of the femur	Sacral plexus (S1, S2)	• External rotation, abduction, and extension of the hip joint • Stabilizes the hip joint
Obturator internus	Inner surface of the obturator membrane and its bony boundaries	Medial surface of the greater trochanter		External rotation, adduction, and extension of the hip joint (also active in abduction, depending on the joint's position)
Gemelli	• Gemellus superior: ischial spine • Gemellus inferior: ischial tuberosity	Jointly with obturator internus tendon (medial surface, greater trochanter)	Sacral plexus (L5, S1)	
Quadratus femoris	Lateral border of the ischial tuberosity	Intertrochanteric crest of the femur		External rotation and adduction of the hip joint

Source: From Gilroy AM et al. Atlas of Anatomy. 3rd ed. 2016. Based on: Schuenke M, Schulte E, Schumacher U. THIEME Atlas of Anatomy. General Anatomy and Musculoskeletal System. Illustrations by Voll M and Wesker K. 2nd ed. New York: Thieme Medical Publishers; 2014.

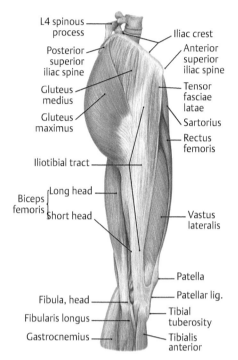

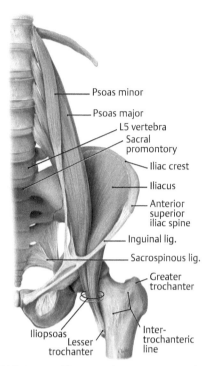

Fig. 11.6 Lateral muscles of the hip, thigh, and gluteal region. Source: From Schuenke M, Schulte E, Schumacher U. THIEME Atlas of Anatomy. General Anatomy and Musculoskeletal System. Illustrations by Voll M and Wesker K. 2nd ed. New York: Thieme Medical Publishers; 2014.

Fig. 11.7 Psoas and iliacus muscles. Source: From Gilroy AM et al. Atlas of Anatomy. 3rd ed. 2016. Based on: Schuenke M, Schulte E, Schumacher U. THIEME Atlas of Anatomy. General Anatomy and Musculoskeletal System. Illustrations by Voll M and Wesker K. 2nd ed. New York: Thieme Medical Publishers; 2014.

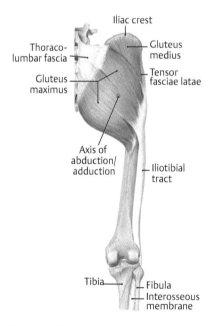

Fig. 11.8 Superficial muscles of the gluteal region. Source: From Schuenke M, Schulte E, Schumacher U. THIEME Atlas of Anatomy. General Anatomy and Musculoskeletal System. Illustrations by Voll M and Wesker K. 2nd ed. New York: Thieme Medical Publishers; 2014.

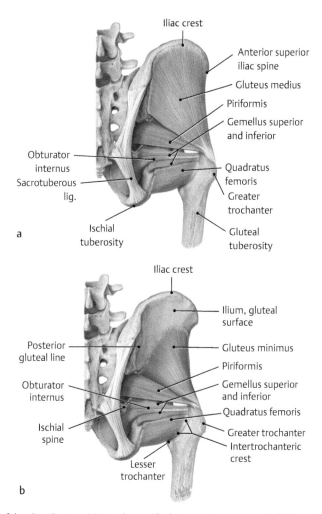

Fig. 11.9 Deep muscles of the gluteal region. (**a**) Deep layer with gluteus maximus removed. (**b**) Deep layer with gluteus maximus and gluteus medius removed. Source: From Schuenke M, Schulte E, Schumacher U. THIEME Atlas of Anatomy. General Anatomy and Musculoskeletal System. Illustrations by Voll M and Wesker K. 2nd ed. New York: Thieme Medical Publishers; 2014.

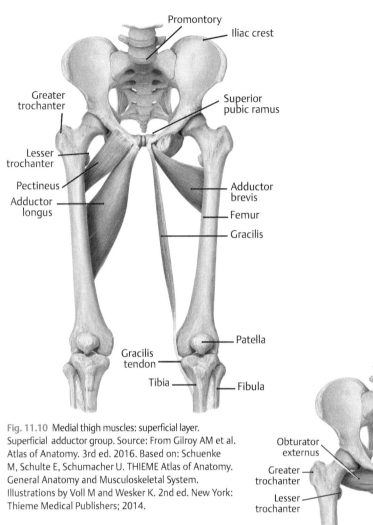

Fig. 11.10 Medial thigh muscles: superficial layer. Superficial adductor group. Source: From Gilroy AM et al. Atlas of Anatomy. 3rd ed. 2016. Based on: Schuenke M, Schulte E, Schumacher U. THIEME Atlas of Anatomy. General Anatomy and Musculoskeletal System. Illustrations by Voll M and Wesker K. 2nd ed. New York: Thieme Medical Publishers; 2014.

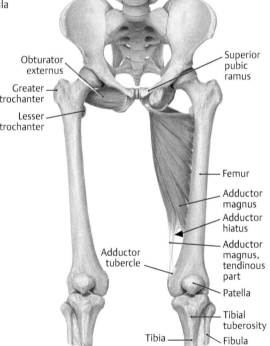

Fig. 11.11 Medial thigh muscles: deep layer. Deep adductor group. Source: From Gilroy AM et al. Atlas of Anatomy. 3rd ed. 2016. Based on: Schuenke M, Schulte E, Schumacher U. THIEME Atlas of Anatomy. General Anatomy and Musculoskeletal System. Illustrations by Voll M and Wesker K. 2nd ed. New York: Thieme Medical Publishers; 2014.

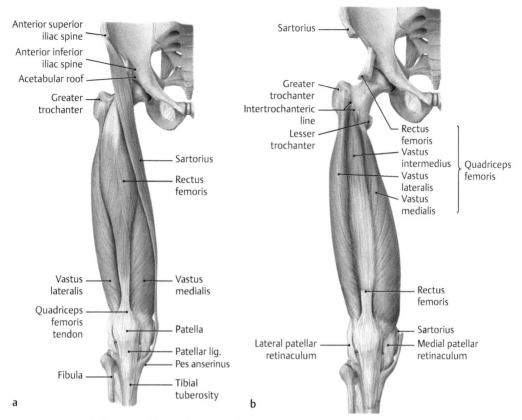

Fig. 11.12 Anterior thigh muscles. (a) Superficial group. (b) Deep group. Removed: Sartorius and rectus femoris. Source: From Schuenke M, Schulte E, Schumacher U. THIEME Atlas of Anatomy. General Anatomy and Musculoskeletal System. Illustrations by Voll M and Wesker K. 2nd ed. New York: Thieme Medical Publishers; 2014.

Table 11.5 Anterior thigh muscles

Muscle		Origin	Insertion	Innervation	Action
Sartorius		Anterior superior iliac spine	Medial to the tibial tuberosity (together with gracilis and semitendinosus)	Femoral n. (L2, L3)	• Hip joint: flexion, abduction, and external rotation • Knee joint: flexion and internal rotation
Quadriceps femoris*	Rectus femoris	Anterior inferior iliac spine, acetabular roof of hip joint	Tibial tuberosity (via patellar lig.)	Femoral n. (L2–L4)	• Hip joint: flexion • Knee joint: extension
	Vastus medialis	Linea aspera (medial lip), intertrochanteric line (distal part)	Both sides of tibial tuberosity on the medial and lateral condyles (via the medial and lateral patellar retinacula)		Knee joint: extension
	Vastus lateralis	Linea aspera (lateral lip), greater trochanter (lateral surface)			
	Vastus intermedius	Femoral shaft (anterior side)	Tibial tuberosity (via patellar lig.)		
	Articularis genus (distal fibers of vastus intermedius)	Anterior side of femoral shaft at level of the suprapatellar recess	Suprapatellar recess of knee joint capsule		Knee joint: extension; prevents entrapment of capsule

*The entire muscle inserts on the tibial tuberosity via the patellar lig.

Source: From Gilroy AM et al. Atlas of Anatomy. 3rd ed. 2016. Based on: Schuenke M, Schulte E, Schumacher U. THIEME Atlas of Anatomy. General Anatomy and Musculoskeletal System. Illustrations by Voll M and Wesker K. 2nd ed. New York: Thieme Medical Publishers; 2014.

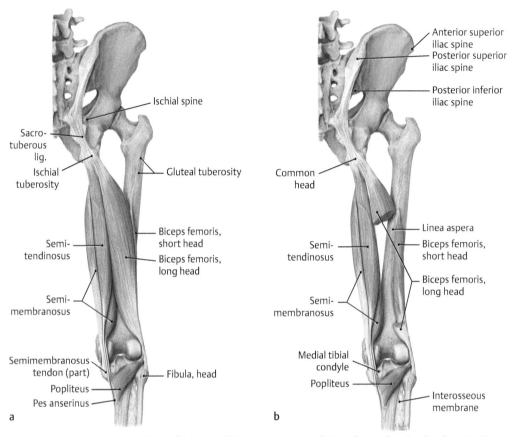

Fig. 11.13 Posterior thigh muscles. (**a**) Superficial group. (**b**) Deep group. Removed: Biceps femoris (long head) and semitendinosus. Source: From Schuenke M, Schulte E, Schumacher U. THIEME Atlas of Anatomy. General Anatomy and Musculoskeletal System. Illustrations by Voll M and Wesker K. 2nd ed. New York: Thieme Medical Publishers; 2014.

Table 11.6 Posterior thigh muscles

Muscle	Origin	Insertion	Innervation	Action
Biceps femoris	Long head: ischial tuberosity, sacrotuberous lig. (common head with semitendinosus)	Head of fibula	Tibial n. (L5–S2)	• Hip joint (long head): extends the hip, stabilizes the pelvis in the sagittal plane • Knee joint: flexion and external rotation
	Short head: lateral lip of the linea aspera in the middle third of the femur		Common fibular n. (L5–S2)	Knee joint: flexion and external rotation
Semimembranosus	Ischial tuberosity	Medial tibial condyle, oblique popliteal lig., popliteus fascia	Tibial n. (L5–S2)	• Hip joint: extends the hip, stabilizes the pelvis in the sagittal plane • Knee joint: flexion and internal rotation
Semitendinosus	Ischial tuberosity and sacrotuberous lig. (common head with long head of biceps femoris)	Medial to the tibial tuberosity in the pes anserinus (along with the tendons of gracilis and sartorius)		

Source: From Gilroy AM et al. Atlas of Anatomy. 3rd ed. 2016. Based on: Schuenke M, Schulte E, Schumacher U. THIEME Atlas of Anatomy. General Anatomy and Musculoskeletal System. Illustrations by Voll M and Wesker K. 2nd ed. New York: Thieme Medical Publishers; 2014.

Muscles of the Leg and Foot

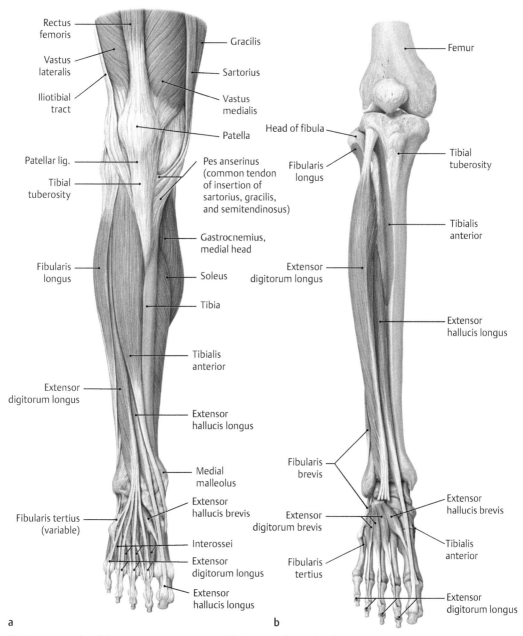

Fig. 11.14 Muscles of the anterior compartment of the leg. (**a**) All muscles shown. (**b**) Removed: Tibialis anterior and fibularis longus; extensor digitorum longus tendons (distal portions). Note: The fibularis tertius is a division of the extensor digitorum longus. Source: From Schuenke M, Schulte E, Schumacher U. THIEME Atlas of Anatomy. General Anatomy and Musculoskeletal System. Illustrations by Voll M and Wesker K. 2nd ed. New York: Thieme Medical Publishers; 2014.

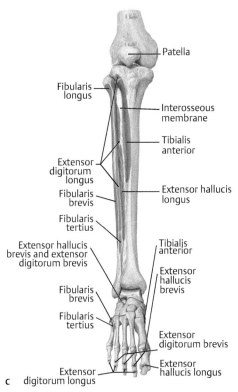

Fig. 11.14 (*Continued*) Muscles of the anterior compartment of the leg. (**c**) Removed: All muscles. Source: From Schuenke M, Schulte E, Schumacher U. THIEME Atlas of Anatomy. General Anatomy and Musculoskeletal System. Illustrations by Voll M and Wesker K. 2nd ed. New York: Thieme Medical Publishers; 2014.

Table 11.7 Anterior compartment

Muscle	Origin	Insertion	Innervation	Action
Tibialis anterior	Tibia (upper two thirds of the lateral surface), interosseous membrane, and superficial crural fascia (highest part)	Medial cuneiform (medial and plantar surface), first metatarsal (medial base)	Deep fibular n. (L4, L5)	• Talocrural joint: dorsiflexion • Subtalar joint: inversion (supination)
Extensor hallucis longus	Fibula (middle third of the medial surface), interosseous membrane	1st toe (at the dorsal aponeurosis at the base of its distal phalanx)	Deep fibular n. (L4, L5)	• Talocrural joint: dorsiflexion • Subtalar joint: active in both eversion and inversion (pronation/supination), depending on the initial position of the foot • Extends the MTP and IP joints of the big toe
Extensor digitorum longus	Fibula (head and medial surface), tibia (lateral condyle), and interosseous membrane	2nd to 5th toes (at the dorsal aponeuroses at the bases of the distal phalanges)	Deep fibular n. (L4, L5)	• Talocrural joint: dorsiflexion • Subtalar joint: eversion (pronation) • Extends the MTP and IP joints of the 2nd to 5th toes
Fibularis tertius	Distal fibula (anterior border)	5th metatarsal (base)	Deep fibular n. (L4, L5)	• Talocrural joint: dorsiflexion • Subtalar joint: eversion (pronation)

Abbreviations: IP, interphalangeal; MTP, metatarsophalangeal.

Source: From Gilroy AM et al. Atlas of Anatomy. 3rd ed. 2016. Based on: Schuenke M, Schulte E, Schumacher U. THIEME Atlas of Anatomy. General Anatomy and Musculoskeletal System. Illustrations by Voll M and Wesker K. 2nd ed. New York: Thieme Medical Publishers; 2014.

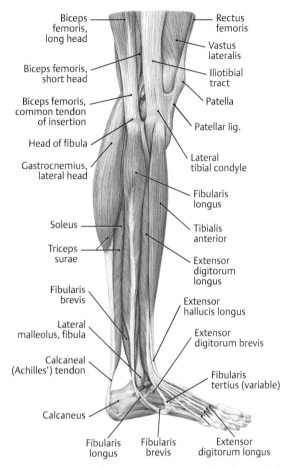

Fig. 11.15 Muscles of the lateral compartment of the leg. Source: From Schuenke M, Schulte E, Schumacher U. THIEME Atlas of Anatomy. General Anatomy and Musculoskeletal System. Illustrations by Voll M and Wesker K. 2nd ed. New York: Thieme Medical Publishers; 2014.

Table 11.8 Lateral compartment

Muscle	Origin	Insertion	Innervation	Action
Fibularis longus	Fibula (head and proximal two thirds of the lateral surface, arising partly from the intermuscular septa)	Medial cuneiform (plantar side), 1st metatarsal (base)	Superficial fibular n. (L5, S1)	• Talocrural joint: plantar flexion • Subtalar joint: eversion (pronation) • Supports the transverse arch of the foot
Fibularis brevis	Fibula (distal half of the lateral surface), intermuscular septa	5th metatarsal (tuberosity at the base, with an occasional division to the dorsal aponeurosis of the 5th toe)		• Talocrural joint: plantar flexion • Subtalar joint: eversion (pronation)

Source: From Gilroy AM et al. Atlas of Anatomy. 3rd ed. 2016. Based on: Schuenke M, Schulte E, Schumacher U. THIEME Atlas of Anatomy. General Anatomy and Musculoskeletal System. Illustrations by Voll M and Wesker K. 2nd ed. New York: Thieme Medical Publishers; 2014.

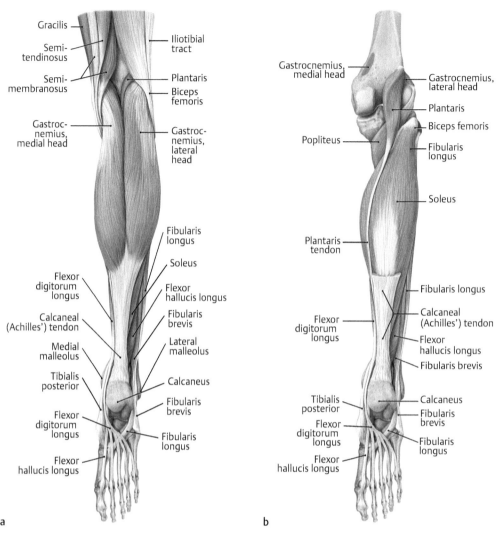

Fig. 11.16 Muscles of the posterior compartment of the leg. (**a**) Note: The bulge of the calf is produced mainly by the triceps surae (soleus and the two heads of the gastrocnemius). (**b**) *Removed:* Gastrocnemius (both heads). Source: From Schuenke M, Schulte E, Schumacher U. THIEME Atlas of Anatomy. General Anatomy and Musculoskeletal System. Illustrations by Voll M and Wesker K. 2nd ed. New York: Thieme Medical Publishers; 2014.

Table 11.9 Superficial flexors of the posterior compartment

Muscle		Origin	Insertion	Innervation	Action
Triceps surae	Gastrocnemius	Femur (medial head: superior posterior part of the medial femoral condyle. lateral head: lateral surface of lateral femoral condyle)	Calcaneal tuberosity via the calcaneal (Achilles') tendon	Tibial n. (S1, S2)	• Talocrural joint: plantar flexion when knee is extended (gastrocnemius) • Knee joint: flexion (gastrocnemius) • Talocrural joint: plantar flexion (soleus)
	Soleus	Fibula (head and neck, posterior surface), tibia (soleal line via a tendinous arch)			
Plantaris		Femur (lateral epicondyle, proximal to lateral head of gastrocnemius)	Calcaneal tuberosity		Negligible; may act with gastrocnemius in plantar flexion

Source: From Gilroy AM et al. Atlas of Anatomy. 3rd ed. 2016. Based on: Schuenke M, Schulte E, Schumacher U. THIEME Atlas of Anatomy. General Anatomy and Musculoskeletal System. Illustrations by Voll M and Wesker K. 2nd ed. New York: Thieme Medical Publishers; 2014.

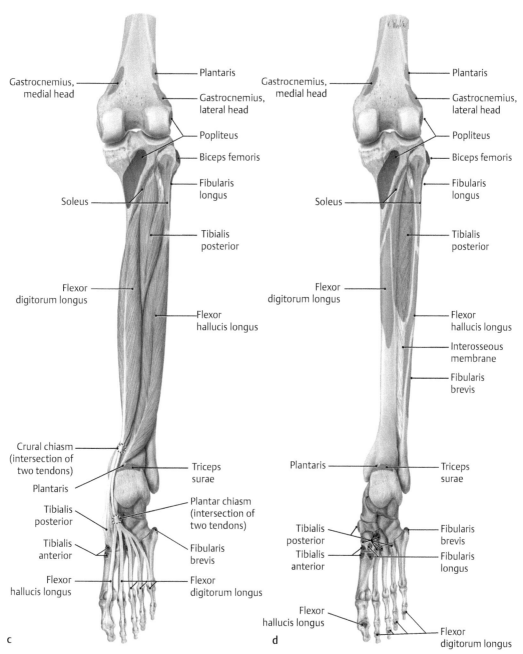

Gastrocnemius, medial head

Plantaris

Gastrocnemius, lateral head

Popliteus

Biceps femoris

Fibularis longus

Soleus

Tibialis posterior

Flexor digitorum longus

Flexor hallucis longus

Crural chiasm (intersection of two tendons)

Plantaris

Triceps surae

Tibialis posterior

Plantar chiasm (intersection of two tendons)

Tibialis anterior

Fibularis brevis

Flexor hallucis longus

Flexor digitorum longus

c

Gastrocnemius, medial head

Plantaris

Gastrocnemius, lateral head

Popliteus

Biceps femoris

Fibularis longus

Soleus

Tibialis posterior

Flexor digitorum longus

Flexor hallucis longus

Interosseous membrane

Fibularis brevis

Plantaris

Triceps surae

Tibialis posterior

Fibularis brevis

Tibialis anterior

Fibularis longus

Flexor hallucis longus

Flexor digitorum longus

d

Fig. 11.16 (*Continued*) Muscles of the posterior compartment of the leg. (**c**) *Removed:* Triceps surae, plantaris, popliteus, fibularis longus, and fibularis brevis muscles. (**d**) *Removed:* All muscles. Source: From Schuenke M, Schulte E, Schumacher U. THIEME Atlas of Anatomy. General Anatomy and Musculoskeletal System. Illustrations by Voll M and Wesker K. 2nd ed. New York: Thieme Medical Publishers; 2014.

Table 11.10 Deep flexors of the posterior compartment

Muscle	Origin	Insertion	Innervation	Action
Tibialis posterior	Interosseous membrane, adjacent borders of tibia and fibula	Navicular tuberosity; cuneiforms (medial, intermediate, and lateral); 2nd to 4th metatarsals (bases)	Tibial n. (L4, L5)	• Talocrural joint: plantar flexion • Subtalar joint: inversion (supination) • Supports the longitudinal and transverse arches
Flexor digitorum longus	Tibia (middle third of posterior surface)	2nd to 5th distal phalanges (bases)		• Talocrural joint: plantar flexion • Subtalar joint: inversion (supination) • MTP and IP joints of the 2nd to 5th toes: plantar flexion
Flexor hallucis longus	Fibula (distal two thirds of posterior surface), adjacent interosseous membrane	1st distal phalanx (base)	Tibial n. (L5–S2)	• Talocrural joint: plantar flexion • Subtalar joint: inversion (supination) • MTP and IP joints of the 1st toe: plantar flexion • Supports the medial longitudinal arch
Popliteus	Lateral femoral condyle, posterior horn of the lateral meniscus	Posterior tibial surface (above the origin at the soleus)	Tibial n. (L4–S1)	Knee joint: flexes and unlocks the knee by internally rotating the femur on the fixed tibia 5°

Abbreviations: IP, interphalangeal; MTP, metatarsophalangeal.

Source: From Gilroy AM et al. Atlas of Anatomy. 3rd ed. 2016. Based on: Schuenke M, Schulte E, Schumacher U. THIEME Atlas of Anatomy. General Anatomy and Musculoskeletal System. Illustrations by Voll M and Wesker K. 2nd ed. New York: Thieme Medical Publishers; 2014.

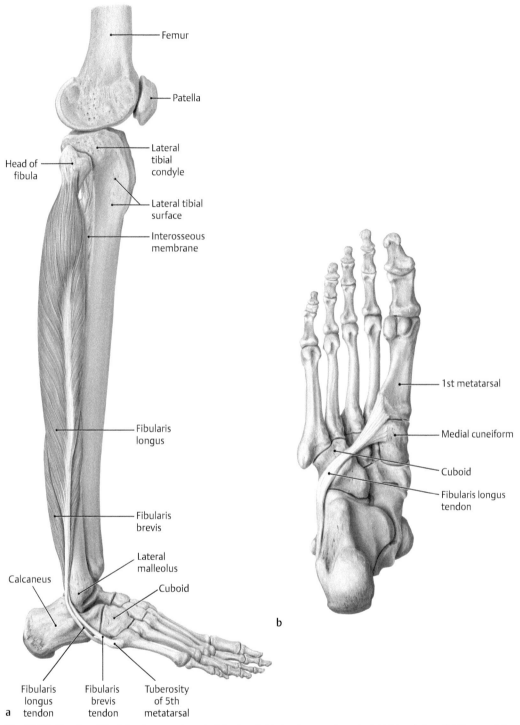

Fig. 11.17 Muscles of the lateral compartment of the leg. (**a**) Lateral compartment, right lateral view. (**b**) Course of the fibularis longus tendon, plantar view. Source: From Schuenke M, Schulte E, Schumacher U. THIEME Atlas of Anatomy. General Anatomy and Musculoskeletal System. Illustrations by Voll M and Wesker K. 2nd ed. New York: Thieme Medical Publishers; 2014.

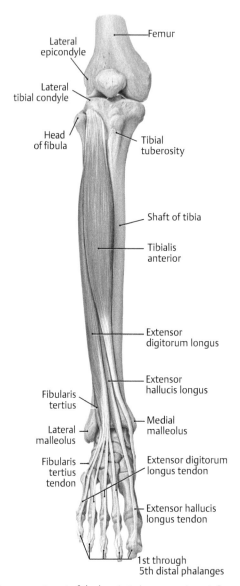

Fig. 11.18 Muscles of the anterior compartment of the leg. Anterior compartment. Source: From Schuenke M, Schulte E, Schumacher U. THIEME Atlas of Anatomy. General Anatomy and Musculoskeletal System. Illustrations by Voll M and Wesker K. 2nd ed. New York: Thieme Medical Publishers; 2014.

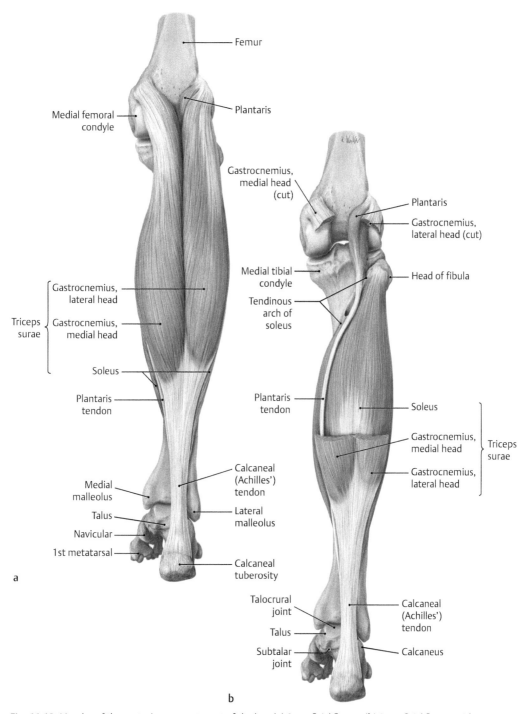

Fig. 11.19 Muscles of the posterior compartment of the leg. (**a**) Superficial flexors (**b**) Superficial flexors with gastrocnemius Removed (portions of medial and lateral heads). Source: From Schuenke M, Schulte E, Schumacher U. THIEME Atlas of Anatomy. General Anatomy and Musculoskeletal System. Illustrations by Voll M and Wesker K. 2nd ed. New York: Thieme Medical Publishers; 2014.

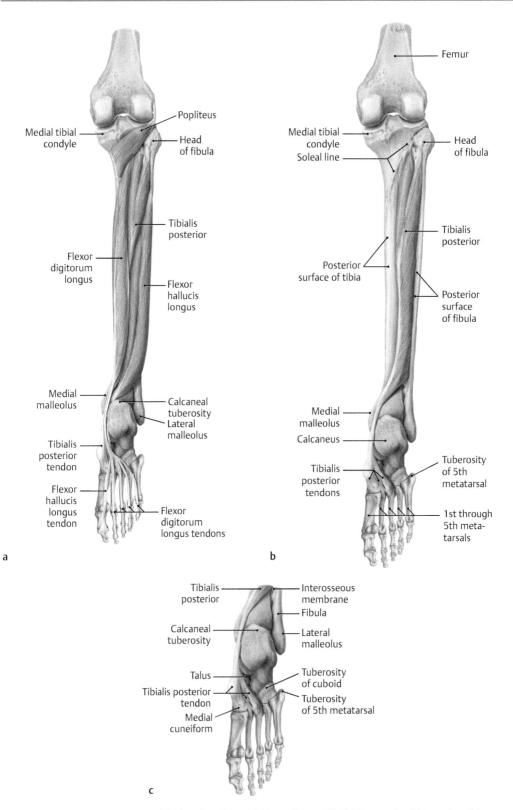

Fig. 11.20 Posterior compartment of the leg: deep flexors. (**a**) Deep flexors. (**b**) Tibialis posterior. (**c**) Insertion of the tibialis posterior. Source: From Schuenke M, Schulte E, Schumacher U. THIEME Atlas of Anatomy. General Anatomy and Musculoskeletal System. Illustrations by Voll M and Wesker K. 2nd ed. New York: Thieme Medical Publishers; 2014.

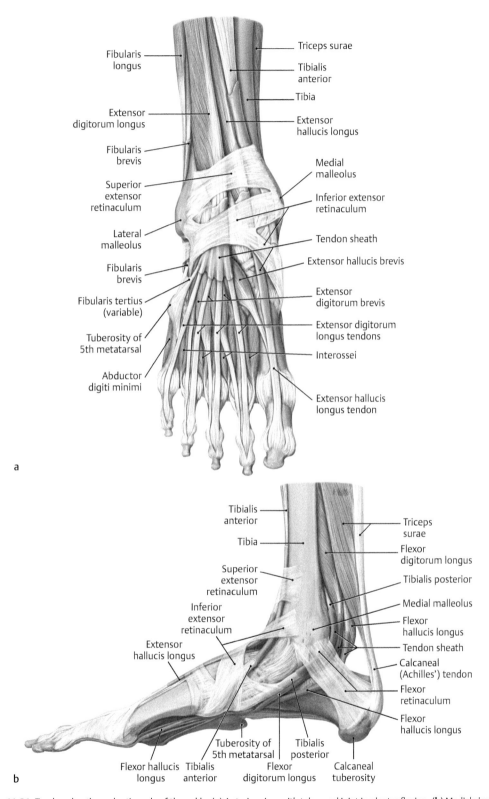

Fibularis longus

Triceps surae

Tibialis anterior

Tibia

Extensor digitorum longus

Extensor hallucis longus

Fibularis brevis

Medial malleolus

Superior extensor retinaculum

Inferior extensor retinaculum

Lateral malleolus

Tendon sheath

Fibularis brevis

Extensor hallucis brevis

Fibularis tertius (variable)

Extensor digitorum brevis

Tuberosity of 5th metatarsal

Extensor digitorum longus tendons

Interossei

Abductor digiti minimi

Extensor hallucis longus tendon

a

Tibialis anterior

Tibia

Triceps surae

Flexor digitorum longus

Superior extensor retinaculum

Tibialis posterior

Inferior extensor retinaculum

Medial malleolus

Extensor hallucis longus

Flexor hallucis longus

Tendon sheath

Calcaneal (Achilles') tendon

Flexor retinaculum

Flexor hallucis longus

Tuberosity of 5th metatarsal

Tibialis posterior

Flexor hallucis longus

Tibialis anterior

Flexor digitorum longus

Calcaneal tuberosity

b

Fig. 11.21 Tendon sheaths and retinacula of the ankle. (a) Anterior view with talocrural joint in plantar flexion. (b) Medial view. Source: From Schuenke M, Schulte E, Schumacher U. THIEME Atlas of Anatomy. General Anatomy and Musculoskeletal System. Illustrations by Voll M and Wesker K. 2nd ed. New York: Thieme Medical Publishers; 2014.

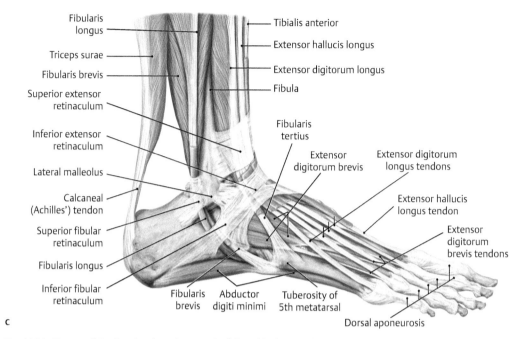

Fibularis longus

Triceps surae

Fibularis brevis

Superior extensor retinaculum

Inferior extensor retinaculum

Lateral malleolus

Calcaneal (Achilles') tendon

Superior fibular retinaculum

Fibularis longus

Inferior fibular retinaculum

Tibialis anterior

Extensor hallucis longus

Extensor digitorum longus

Fibula

Fibularis tertius

Extensor digitorum brevis

Extensor digitorum longus tendons

Extensor hallucis longus tendon

Extensor digitorum brevis tendons

Fibularis brevis

Abductor digiti minimi

Tuberosity of 5th metatarsal

Dorsal aponeurosis

c

Fig. 11.21 (*Continued*) Tendon sheaths and retinacula of the ankle. (**c**) Lateral view. Source: From Schuenke M, Schulte E, Schumacher U. THIEME Atlas of Anatomy. General Anatomy and Musculoskeletal System. Illustrations by Voll M and Wesker K. 2nd ed. New York: Thieme Medical Publishers; 2014.

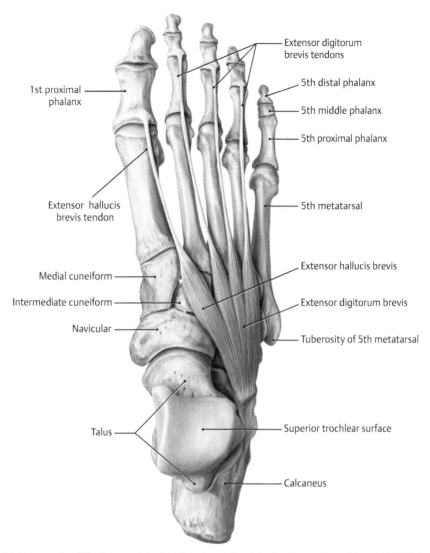

Fig. 11.22 Intrinsic muscles of the dorsum of the foot. Dorsal muscles of the foot. Source: From Schuenke M, Schulte E, Schumacher U. THIEME Atlas of Anatomy. General Anatomy and Musculoskeletal System. Illustrations by Voll M and Wesker K. 2nd ed. New York: Thieme Medical Publishers; 2014.

Table 11.11 Intrinsic muscles of the dorsum of the foot

Muscle	Origin	Insertion	Innervation	Action
Extensor digitorum brevis	Calcaneus (dorsal surface)	2nd to 4th toes (at dorsal aponeuroses and bases of the middle phalanges)	Deep fibular n. (L5, S1)	Extension of the MTP and PIP joints of the 2nd to 4th toes
Extensor hallucis brevis		1st toe (at dorsal aponeurosis and proximal phalanx)		Extension of the MTP joints of the 1st toe

Abbreviations: MTP, metatarsophalangeal; PIP, proximal interphalangeal.

Source: From Gilroy AM et al. Atlas of Anatomy. 3rd ed. 2016. Based on: Schuenke M, Schulte E, Schumacher U. THIEME Atlas of Anatomy. General Anatomy and Musculoskeletal System. Illustrations by Voll M and Wesker K. 2nd ed. New York: Thieme Medical Publishers; 2014.

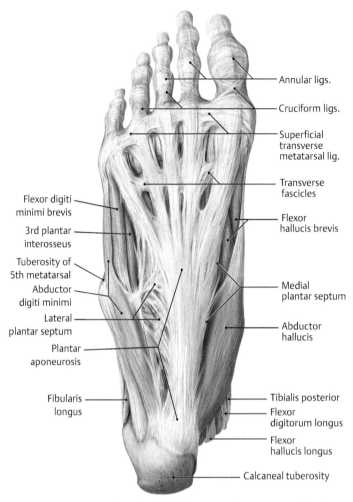

Fig. 11.23 Plantar aponeurosis. Source: From Schuenke M, Schulte E, Schumacher U. THIEME Atlas of Anatomy. General Anatomy and Musculoskeletal System. Illustrations by Voll M and Wesker K. 2nd ed. New York: Thieme Medical Publishers; 2014.

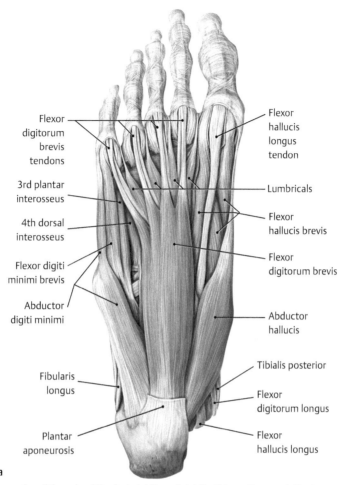

Fig. 11.24 Intrinsic muscles of the sole of the foot. (**a**) Superficial (first) layer. Removed: Plantar aponeurosis, including the superficial transverse metacarpal ligament. Source: From Schuenke M, Schulte E, Schumacher U. THIEME Atlas of Anatomy. General Anatomy and Musculoskeletal System. Illustrations by Voll M and Wesker K. 2nd ed. New York: Thieme Medical Publishers; 2014.

Table 11.12 Superficial intrinsic muscles of the sole of the foot

Muscle	Origin	Insertion	Innervation	Action
Abductor hallucis	Calcaneal tuberosity (medial process); flexor retinaculum, plantar aponeurosis	1st toe (base of proximal phalanx via the medial sesamoid)	Medial plantar n. (S1, S2)	• 1st MTP joint: flexion and abduction of the 1st toe • Supports the longitudinal arch
Flexor digitorum brevis	Calcaneal tuberosity (medial tubercle), plantar aponeurosis	2nd to 5th toes (sides of middle phalanges)		• Flexes the MTP and PIP joints of the 2nd to 5th toes • Supports the longitudinal arch
Abductor digiti minimi		5th toe (base of proximal phalanx), 5th metatarsal (at tuberosity)	Lateral plantar n. (S1–S3)	• Flexes the MTP joint of the 5th toe • Abducts the 5th toe • Supports the longitudinal arch

Abbreviations: MTP, metatarsophalangeal; PIP, proximal interphalangeal.

Source: From Gilroy AM et al. Atlas of Anatomy. 3rd ed. 2016. Based on: Schuenke M, Schulte E, Schumacher U. THIEME Atlas of Anatomy. General Anatomy and Musculoskeletal System. Illustrations by Voll M and Wesker K. 2nd ed. New York: Thieme Medical Publishers; 2014.

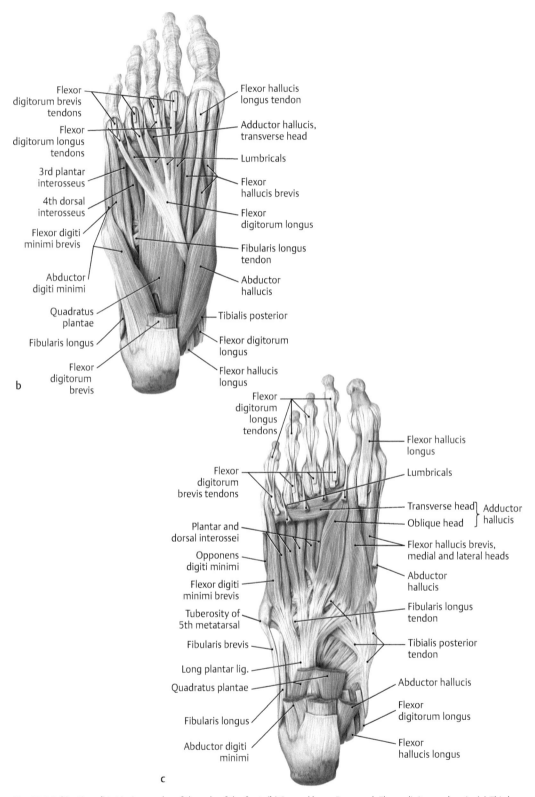

Flexor digitorum brevis tendons

Flexor digitorum longus tendons

3rd plantar interosseus

4th dorsal interosseus

Flexor digiti minimi brevis

Abductor digiti minimi

Quadratus plantae

Fibularis longus

Flexor digitorum brevis

Flexor hallucis longus tendon

Adductor hallucis, transverse head

Lumbricals

Flexor hallucis brevis

Flexor digitorum longus

Fibularis longus tendon

Abductor hallucis

Tibialis posterior

Flexor digitorum longus

Flexor hallucis longus

b

Flexor digitorum longus tendons

Flexor digitorum brevis tendons

Plantar and dorsal interossei

Opponens digiti minimi

Flexor digiti minimi brevis

Tuberosity of 5th metatarsal

Fibularis brevis

Long plantar lig.

Quadratus plantae

Fibularis longus

Abductor digiti minimi

Flexor hallucis longus

Lumbricals

Transverse head ⎫ Adductor
Oblique head   ⎰ hallucis

Flexor hallucis brevis, medial and lateral heads

Abductor hallucis

Fibularis longus tendon

Tibialis posterior tendon

Abductor hallucis

Flexor digitorum longus

Flexor hallucis longus

c

Fig. 11.24 (*Continued*) Intrinsic muscles of the sole of the foot. (**b**) Second layer. Removed: Flexor digitorum brevis. (**c**) Third layer. Removed: Abductor digiti minimi, abductor hallucis, quadratus plantae, lumbricals, and tendons of insertion of the flexors digitorum and hallucis longus. Source: From Schuenke M, Schulte E, Schumacher U. THIEME Atlas of Anatomy. General Anatomy and Musculoskeletal System. Illustrations by Voll M and Wesker K. 2nd ed. New York: Thieme Medical Publishers; 2014.

Table 11.13 Deep intrinsic muscles of the sole of the foot

Muscle	Origin	Insertion	Innervation	Action
Quadratus plantae	Calcaneal tuberosity (medial and plantar borders on plantar side)	Flexor digitorum longus tendon (lateral border)	Lateral plantar n. (S1–S3)	Redirects and augments the pull of flexor digitorum longus
Lumbricals (four muscles)	Flexor digitorum longus tendons (medial borders)	2nd to 5th toes (at dorsal aponeuroses)	1st lumbrical: medial plantar n. (S2, S3) 2nd to 4th lumbrical: lateral plantar n. (S2, S3)	• Flexes the MTP joints of 2nd to 5th toes • Extension of IP joints of 2nd to 5th toes • Adducts 2nd to 5th toes toward the big toe
Flexor hallucis brevis	Cuboid, lateral cuneiforms, and plantar calcaneocuboid lig.	1st toe (at base of proximal phalanx via medial and lateral sesamoids)	Medial head: medial plantar n. (S1, S2) Lateral head: lateral plantar n. (S1, S2)	• Flexes the first MTP joint • Supports the longitudinal arch
Adductor hallucis	Oblique head: 2nd to 4th metatarsals (at bases) cuboid and lateral cuneiforms Transverse head: MTP joints of 3rd to 5th toes, deep transverse metatarsal lig.	1st proximal phalanx (at base, by a common tendon via the lateral sesamoid)	Lateral plantar n., deep branch (S2, S3)	• Flexes the first MTP joint • Adducts big toe • Transverse head: supports transverse arch • Oblique head: supports longitudinal arch
Flexor digiti minimi brevis	5th metatarsal (base), long plantar lig.	5th toe (base of proximal phalanx)	Lateral plantar n., superficial branch (S2, S3)	Flexes the MTP joint of the little toe
Opponens digiti minimi*	Long plantar lig.; fibularis longus (at plantar tendon sheath)	5th metatarsal		Pulls 5th metatarsal in plantar and medial direction
Plantar interossei (three muscles)	3rd to 5th metatarsals (medial border)	3rd to 5th toes (medial base of proximal phalanx)		• Flexes the MTP joints of 3rd to 5th toes • Extension of IP joints of 3rd to 5th toes • Adducts 3rd to 5th toes toward 2nd toe
Dorsal interossei (four muscles)	1st to 5th metatarsals (by two heads on opposing sides)	1st interosseus: 2nd proximal phalanx (medial base) 2nd to 4th interossei: 2nd to 4th proximal phalanges (lateral base), 2nd to 4th toes (at dorsal aponeuroses)	Lateral plantar n. (S2, S3)	• Flexes the MTP joints of 2nd to 4th toes • Extension of IP joints of 2nd to 4th toes • Abducts 3rd and 4th toes from 2nd toe

Abbreviations: IP, interphalangeal; MTP, metatarsophalangeal. *May be absent.

Source: From Gilroy AM et al. Atlas of Anatomy. 3rd ed. 2016. Based on: Schuenke M, Schulte E, Schumacher U. THIEME Atlas of Anatomy. General Anatomy and Musculoskeletal System. Illustrations by Voll M and Wesker K. 2nd ed. New York: Thieme Medical Publishers; 2014.

Index

Note: Page numbers set in *f* and *t* indicate figures and tables respectively.